The Warrior's Path
Living Yoga's Ten Codes

Derek Beres

For bibliography visit otbpublishing.com/thewarriorspath

Front and back cover photographs: Joshua Nelson

To Philip Steir, for joining me on this journey.

CONTENTS

We are potentially moral animals—which is more than any other animal can say—but we aren't naturally moral animals. To be moral animals, we must realize how thoroughly we aren't.

Robert Wright, *The Moral Animal*

Awakening does not mean an end to difficulty; it means a change in the way those difficulties are met.

Mark Epstein, *The Trauma of Everyday Life*

INTRODUCTION

WHILE WE MOVE THE BODY, we are not the body. We are so much more than this meaty casing of flesh and muscle, synaptic connections and blood-soaked organs. Through yoga we transcend so the body will no longer be a hindrance.

You walk out of the studio, confused as to who the *you* is propelling these legs forward, pupils dilated with sunbeams, a sordid breeze of springtime and exhaust fumes assaulting your nostrils. If you are not your body, what was just speeding through hundreds of postures over the last ninety minutes?

Place all your weight on your right foot and straighten your left leg forward to a ninety-degree angle. Lock your standing leg as you pull your face toward your shin.

The legs that aren't yours suddenly turn gelatinous. It's 100 degrees in a room that smells like a hospital floor. Sixty people crowd you. There is one shower. You know you're not going to get there first or, most likely, at all.

Ad Guray Nameh, Jugad Guray Nameh, Sat Guray Nameh, Siri Guru Devay Nameh.

For forty-five minutes now. The chant isn't bothering you. The fact that your arms—*are these really your arms?*—have been waving wildly above your head the entire time takes precedence. You were told these words had to do with bowing, but you haven't leaned forward once. Here there is *no* shower.

Great stress reliever. Tones the abdomens and thighs. Makes your ass look great in a bathing suit. Introduces you to the Divine. Rids you of the body. Introduces you to the body. The only way to true enlightenment.

1

Welcome to yoga.

"IF THE WORD 'YOGA' *means* many things," writes the great historian of religions, Mircea Eliade, "that is because Yoga *is* many things." This seeming virtue—a widespread practice as flexible as the postures defining much of its modern incarnation—is also a vice. As Indian scholar and chemist I.K. Taimni writes regarding yoga, "There is no subject which is so much wrapped up in mystery and on which one can write whatever one likes without any risk of being proved wrong."

Being wrong is not a primary concern of mine in this book. I have no intention of defining what yoga *is* or *is not*. The recurring sentiment on social media and in classes that any one style or lineage has ownership of yoga is preposterous and in no way historically accurate. As Taoists say, many rivers lead to one ocean. This does not imply yoga is without a foundation, however.

Yoga serves a variety of functions for a broad range of people. Since I began studying Indian texts in 1993, and, six years later, yoga postures, I've been a mutt, checking out this style, moving that way. I'm too fascinated with the myriad means in which we express our bodies to restrict a process and discipline as great as yoga to one singular meaning.

Postures are what most people associate with yoga these days. Yogis who dedicate their lives to it are sometimes frustrated by this phenomenon. I do not view it as a bad thing. With soaring obesity rates, a growing dependence on pharmaceuticals, and a dizzying array of nutritional misinformation packaged as science, anything helping us live healthier, more productive lifestyles is a good thing. I'm not going to explore a wide range of exercise formats in these pages. There are many books already offering this. I want to investigate something else entirely.

Yoga has become a big business in our country, and when dollar signs appear all sorts of definitions pop up. According to a 2012 study conducted by NAMASTA, Americans spend $10.3 billion on a variety of services related to yoga each year, nearly double the amount spent four years prior. The very term, as Taimni states, becomes a catchall; it means whatever the person talking about it wants it to mean. On numerous occasions I've heard someone claim yoga is 'whatever you want it to be.' If yoga can be anything, then really it's nothing. It has no meaning, no morality, no consequences, and therefore no value.

Yoga does not conveniently fit into a desired package without losing credibility. As inventive as some teachers have made the physical practice, groundwork is necessary, a container to hold the discipline together. Fortunately a man named Patanjali penned the *Yoga Sutras* around the second century CE to give generations of practitioners a platform to work with. Little is known of him; there were at least three Patanjalis at that time, and none of them might be the one who scribed the *Sutras*. Regardless, his eight limbs have become the requisite framework modern American yoga is, at least philosophically, related to.

This book focuses on the first two rungs of Patanjali's ladder. The *yamas* and *niyamas*, or yogic 'do's' and 'do not's,' have long served as the moral foundation at the base of this discipline. In America we usually skip ahead to the third rung, *asanas* (postures), and, if all goes well, progress to the other five, all of which deal with meditation and turning inward on some level. Traditionally a yogi was not allowed to begin with postures—and postures meant sitting for meditation, not the aerobic exercise movements we think of today (*asana* originally meant 'seat'). As religious scholar Karen Armstrong writes, "The yogin had to undergo a long period of preparation. He was not allowed to perform a single yogic exercise until he had completed an extensive moral training. The aspirant began by observing the yamas ("prohibitions")... The preparatory program also demanded the mastery of certain bodily and psychic disciplines (niyama)."

In America we posture without setting the stage, confusing some in regards to the overall power of yoga. The poses become more about Instagram handstands and mountaintop mudras than right action and thinking. While I am a big fan of the movement practice—I have made my living teaching group classes for over a decade—I feel it important to first stand upon the bedrock. Not only does it help us understand yoga better; putting to practice the ethical restraints and moral sentiments teaches us how to relate to others and strengthens our relationship to the planet that has birthed us.

This sounds like a tall order, for good reason. There are many cultural nuances separating us from other nations. And yet ethics, while socially relative, unseats the more esoteric strains of spiritual practices. Most forms of religion and spiritual philosophies are similar from a moral perspective: treat others how you'd like to be treated; don't steal; don't cheat, sexually or socially; study your actions, how you carry yourself in society. Humans are similar in how we enjoy being treated; we are from different universes when it comes to metaphysics. How we got *here*, *who* we are and *how* we were made are not especially important questions if our aim is to live a more fulfilled and compassionate life. How we relate to others, our relationship to the world beyond us, and how we act *are* relevant and, to one degree or another, addressed in Patanjali's ingenious compilation of ideas.

Ethics, however, is not the reason most Americans practice yoga. The top five motivations for getting on the mat have nothing to do with the moral dimension: flexibility, general conditioning, stress relief, improving overall health, and physical fitness top the list. We practice yoga to better ourselves in some capacity. Very rarely do others come to mind, save a growing number of husbands entering the studio to relate to their wives—a great trend, for sure. If, by extension, being a better person extends to how we treat others, we have found an unintended though highly appreciated byproduct.

This focus on self should not shock us. Our nation values individual liberties over all else. Companies market to this peculiar evolution of our tribal origins. Freedom of the individual trumps sustainability of the community. Only when resources are so scarce or a local tragedy occurs do we remember the role of *we* among neighbors. In this sense it's hard to imagine other people (or the earth) being an inspiration for yoga. Fortunately once one begins practicing they see a bigger picture.

The very term 'morals' seems outdated, even though it underlies our emergence as a species. To this day I often associate a moral lifestyle with fundamental religious values. The idea triggers many, especially those 'recovering' from the faith of their youth. Being told what we cannot do inspires us to do exactly that. By the time we reach adulthood and reconsider our youthful rebellion in pursuit of a more stable lifestyle, the possibility of changing how we live immediately sets us off. The morals we practice by this time are often the morals we stick with.

This is because human beings are more reactive than proactive. The slightest implication that we might be wrong forces us into a quick crisis. Our *samskāras*, or mental imprints, are well defined by the time we enter our twenties. Breaking habitual patterns is a daunting prospect.

Yet this was the intention of yogic principles in the first place: to usurp your assumptions of yourself and introduce you to a much richer realm of possibilities. While the earliest recorded sketches usually dealt with transcending the body—unsurprising considering these yogis were warriors in armed engagements confronting death on a regular basis—around the sixth century CE yogis claimed nonviolence to be the clarion call of their practice. This social trend was more recently promoted by Mohandas K. Gandhi, the lawyer-turned-sage who treated the great battle of the *Bhagavad Gītā* as a metaphor for the inner struggle every human wages within himself. Today yoga instructors usually travel this track, treating the literature of early thinkers as symbolic gestures aimed at our highest good.

We're born with a sense of morals. Evolution has prepared us with a handy ethical map inside of our brains. This mapping is subject to cultural and social norms, however. And as with all maps, it is not the terrain. I'll be exploring brain maps and other neural functions throughout this book, as I've spent the least few years developing a national program called Flow Play for Equinox Fitness. Alongside my colleague Philip Steir, we've investigated the intersection of yoga, music and neuroscience. He is responsible for discovering a good amount of neural research within these pages.

Some of the information might surprise you, as neuroscience reveals counterintuitive truths in regards to how our brains operate. It is important to remember that exploring aspects of developmental psychology and evolutionary history does not necessarily condone what is being discussed. It's like an oncologist explaining the mechanisms of cancer. He is not saying that the disease is inherently good or claiming that its origins imply unchangeable results. The opposite is true: he is trying to understand it to change it.

This is the genius of yoga. We study ourselves honestly and thoroughly to become the best possible person we can be. In my own life and practice, yoga has long served this role. I stress my body through movement to alleviate stress. I test the boundaries of my emotions to become more fully attuned to my emotional body. I challenge my beliefs to discover what other possibilities exist. This does not necessarily change my mind, though sometimes it does. Flexibility comes in many forms. Besides, debating one aspect of a complex situation is useless if you cannot at least understand where your opponent comes from. Otherwise you're just shouting without listening, a practice that never bears fruit.

Yale University Psychology and Cognitive Science Professor Paul Bloom writes that we are born with a few particular endowments: a moral sense; empathy and compassion; rudimentary senses of fairness and justice. This innate goodness is limited, though, as it applies only to small familial and social circles. When expanding these principles to what today we call the global village, little of this beauty remains. Bloom continues: "We are by nature indifferent, even hostile, to strangers; we are prone toward parochialism and bigotry. Some of our instinctive emotional responses, most notably disgust, spur us to do terrible things, including acts of genocide."

If, as the popular sentiment in modern yoga goes, we are seeking a world in which everyone is 'happy and free,' a lot of work remains. Our innate senses must conspire with the world we live in, one that has, for thousands of generations, been informed by tribalism. Bloom's indifference has precedence. British anthropologist Robin Dunbar noticed a correlation between the size of primate brains and social group size. The top end of stable human relationships is 150 members, which is also the general number our ancestors capped their societies at.

While this helps explain our hostility toward others outside of our group, working together on a mass scale *is* unique to our species. Social psychologist Jonathan Haidt terms this 'groupishness.' Our ability to hunt, build, and defend in large groups greatly aided the preservation and eventual proliferation of our species. The genetic basis for bias is fed by cultural values; our penchant for overriding personal identity in favor of the group balances these gripes and complaints. Haidt phrases it succinctly: "We're born to be righteous, but we have to learn, what, exactly, people like us should be righteous about."

And that might require a shift of perspective. As much as change frightens us, we're doing it all the time. Sometimes we consciously choose to alter something; at other times, we find ourselves in impossible situations we'd never have dreamed of and must completely reorient ourselves. Yoga helps with both of these—it is training and the battle simultaneously. Yoga is a tool to be used during quiet and chaotic moments alike. With the growing field of neuroscience educating us as to how our brains are wired, we know everything about how we think and process information is plastic. We can rewire our synaptic connections at will. This does not make it easy. But it does make almost anything possible.

To accomplish such a herculean task there needs to be integration. A common sentiment I've noticed of late is the separation of spirituality from religion. The former is treated as a personal connection to the 'universe' or whatever benevolent idea is conjured, the latter viewed as dogmatic and inflexible, the antithesis of what draws people to yoga and the flowing philosophies of the East. Religion is treated as a bane and excuse for actual self-reflection. Assigning humanity's ails to a deity wipes our hands clean of responsibility when belief is considered more important than action. Oddly proponents of the so-called spiritual life often make similar errors of judgment dressed in different clothing. Both terms have positive and negative features depending on the motivational direction behind each.

Etymologically 'religion' and 'yoga' essentially mean the same thing: to bind you to something else, to bring you in communion with yourself or a greater energetic pulse throughout the cosmos—or, more realistically, the planet we all inhabit. While I realize the separation is meant to distance one from dogma, I don't think the problem truly lies in semantics to begin with. For example, one cannot truly be born into a religion. They must embody its teachings for the lessons to resonate. The same holds true of spirituality. Intentions mean little if your actions are not in accordance with what you profess to be your belief system. We are aptly able to deceive others; there's an entire history of gurus and priestly charlatans duping their followers. We should hope, if we're being true to the teachings of our chosen discipline, that we would not deceive ourselves. While that sounds like it should be a default setting, in actuality it takes quite an amount of work.

Yoga is no easy path to tread. Yet the teachings seem so natural: stay clean, study yourself, surrender when necessary, be satisfied with who you are. There is nothing particularly groundbreaking in the *yamas* and *niyamas*. Still, putting them into practice is complex and demands a committed rigor, at least until we reach a point where it *feels* natural. A sculptor whittles down rock to reveal the essence of what was already inside, that which we call art. The aim here is to do the same.

The mythologist Joseph Campbell once remarked that religion needs to evolve with each passing generation if it's going to suit the needs of the times. If a belief system does not serve the people it is addressing—if the figureheads are constantly looking backwards for answers instead of peering out at what's right in front of them—that religion becomes irrelevant. This idea is not restricted to Western faiths. Yogis too attempt to apply ancient doctrines without understanding the historical and cultural context, never realizing that the devil—in this case, the *asura*—is in the details.

Over the course of history many forms of yoga emerged to accommodate the varying needs of different human beings: the rigorous demands of philosophical introspection, the ecstatic bliss of devotion, the royal path of total integration. While most of what we do in gyms and studios is an offshoot of Hatha Yoga, this book is an attempt to pinpoint the intersection of *jnana* yoga, the yoga of knowledge, with karma yoga, the yoga of action. Yoga has to work in both directions: the deep inward reflection of our inner terrain fused with an honest outward gaze at the society we've created and our role within it. It can't be all about us and yet, paradoxically, that's where it all begins. We are the result of what we have built, personally and globally. Let us stare inside to find the light we reflect back out.

1 AHIMSA : THE ART OF A KING

IN 1959, HAVING BEING INSPIRED by the writings of Mohandas K. Gandhi, Martin Luther King, Jr. visited India to learn the principles of nonviolent social protest directly from the great thinker's disciples. Invited by Prime Minister Jawaharlal Nehru in 1956, a series of obligations held up the African-American leader. It was not until an assassination attempt nearly took his life two years later that he decided to travel abroad. King was interested in understanding how Gandhi's vision of nonviolence had manifested in his homeland. Little did he know his Montgomery bus boycott had received more attention in Indian newspapers than at home in the United States. He arrived as a hero and was greeted as a brother.

In an article for *Ebony* published upon his return King described the lack of hatred and bitterness in the Indian people, rare in a population that had just experienced profound longstanding violence at the hands of British forces. He was surprised to find friendships between the former occupier and those occupied, attributing it to the principles of nonviolence implemented during Gandhi's time.

King wrote about an experience meeting a group of African students. They believed nonviolence might work in India, though it would not suffice on their continent. They claimed such an agenda was tenable only if the resisters had a potential ally in the occupiers.

9

To this King replied, "True non-violent resistance is not unrealistic submission to evil power. It is rather a courageous confrontation of evil by the power of love, in the faith that it is better to be the recipient of violence than the inflictor of it, since the latter only multiplies the existence of violence and the bitterness in the universe, while the former may develop a shame in the opponent, and thereby bring about a transformation and change of heart."

Submission was not in Gandhi's vocabulary either. While he admitted violence might be necessary in extreme conditions, his writings on *ahimsa* (nonviolence) and peaceful protests continue to resonate around the world. The Salt March he led in 1930 was possibly the most influential nonviolent protest of the twentieth century, directly inspiring King when he was helping organize the bus boycott in 1955.

Gandhi often turned to his favorite volume of karma yoga lessons, the *Bhagavad Gītā*, for insight and guidance. But he learned the true power of *ahimsa* from his father. At age fifteen he stole a piece of gold from his brother. The agony of his deception tore him up. His father was not an especially forgiving man; the youngster could not bring himself to admit his theft. Instead he scribed his confession on a piece of paper, handing it to his father while fearing painful retribution. His father sat on the edge of the bed and cried, never raising a fist. Gandhi attributes his coming clean before being caught as the reason for his father's compassion.

"This was for me an object lesson in Ahimsa. Then I could read in it nothing more than a father's love but today I know that it was pure Ahimsa. When such Ahimsa becomes all-embracing it transforms everything it touches. There is no limit to its power."

At first glance nonviolence is a surprising talking point in the *Gītā*, given that the 700 stanzas honor one of India's fiercest wars. A slim insert inside the much larger *Mahābhārata*, the *Gītā* is a synthesizing of various indigenous philosophies, including Sāmkhya, Yoga, Vedānta and orthodox Brāhmanism. A devotional hymn to the Vaishnava god Krishna, the flute-playing deity—his name means 'puller' as he attracts devotees' hearts to himself, music being one way he accomplishes this—tells the archer Arjuna not to concern himself when slaying his cousins and friends on the battlefield. The young warrior had been experiencing an existential crisis. Krishna informs the distraught bowman that wise men do not mourn for the living or the dead.

A few paragraphs later the writer reveals his true intention: "If you refuse to fight this righteous war, you will be turning aside from your duty. You will be a sinner, and disgraced. People will speak ill of you throughout the ages. To a man who values his honour, that is surely worse than death."

Duty to your clan was more important than individual liberation. While the *Bhagavad Gitā* is today widely considered an allegorical story, at the time service to your tribe trumped self-preservation. In America we are raised to believe personal identity is the epitome if not the *point* of existence. This is a relatively new historical development. The doctrines defining a wide swath of religions—Hinduism, Christianity, Judaism, Islam—were written when loyalty ruled over all. The karma yoga Arjuna was being instructed in demanded service to his clan, not himself. The emotional crossroads he encountered on the battlefield were the result of personal feelings, which must be surrendered for the advancement of the group.

All armed forces depend on group ideology to succeed. By aligning the divinity to his side, the *Gitā*'s writer makes clear what tribe he wanted righteousness to be associated with. We experience a similar bias today when preachers claim that God whips up hurricanes and tornados to punish Americans for accepting homosexuality. As we'll see later, speakers who invoke a sense of disgust in others dehumanize them, making their ridicule and oppression palatable. Tribal leaders have called for the fear and hatred of others throughout history.

The *Gitā* introduces an interesting riddle: How can an army use a spiritual discipline championing nonviolence? The story might have been allegorical, but over the centuries yoga postures, breathing techniques, and meditation have helped real soldiers calm themselves before heading into battle. From the fifteenth century onward, militarized yogis disrupted trade routes across Northern India, "becoming so powerful in the eighteenth century as to be able to challenge the economic and political hegemony of the East India Company," writes yoga scholar Mark Singleton. Today such aggressive behavior challenges what we consider yogic. Regardless of our assumptions, these men were using familiar techniques to fine-tune their emotional intelligence and mental fortitude in accomplishing the tasks at hand, which were very violent indeed.

Whether nineteenth century mercenaries recovering stolen goods from British imperialists or twenty-first century American soldiers attempting to Westernize Middle Eastern countries, the toll taken on warriors is grueling and depleting. Buddhist teacher Michael Stone questions whether mindfulness techniques can truly be of use in ethically suspect initiatives. Is it possible to practice meditation from a tradition that specifically calls for nonviolence if you're using it to kill others? Traditionally, if a prospective student raged around his neighborhood, a respectable teacher would not allow him to partake in yogic training. Is that because it doesn't 'work' or because said teacher was imparting his own caution?

Stone writes, "Mindfulness was not designed as an ethically indeterminate technique. In the yoga and Buddhist traditions, meditation practice has always been grounded in an understanding of causality, or karma: our actions make a difference. If everything we do has an impact, then mindfulness is a deeply political practice, designed to reduce stress and suffering both in our own hearts and in the world of which we are a part. Those two things are not separate."

I agree with Stone that mindfulness *should* be aimed at nonviolence. It's hard to imagine a situation in which meditation and controlled breathing promote murder. Yet it's context: I don't harbor violent feelings in the first place. Just because I don't agree with slaughtering others for the benefit of my tribe doesn't mean the physiological effects of yoga postures and meditation might not have a different result in others. In this sense these techniques are morally benign: you get out what you put in. The health benefits—lower heart rate and blood pressure, greater mental focus and so forth—will be similar. How you utilize those effects varies widely.

It's important to recognize that yoga is not what we want it to be just because we think we're on the right side of the story. War and slaughter are a major reason that we have the right to practice whatever spirituality we desire in America today. Battles have not been waged on our land in quite some time. Other cultures are not so fortunate. What goes on in America is not a reflection of what happens across the planet. I'm not implying we should abandon the quest for a more peaceful world; the bulk of this book argues that we should be doing exactly that. It is important to note, however, that we always have been and always will be a work in progress. We should recognize the historical forces that have helped shape our identity today. It's not pretty, though it's honest.

In fact we are moving toward nonviolence. According to cognitive scientist Steven Pinker we live in the least violent point in recorded history. There are a number of reasons for this. Global trade means countries rely on resources and goods from other nations. Depending on others for oil, ore, and food implies that you're not going to battle the people shipping those goods to your country. Last century's atomic bombs coupled with the frightening power of nuclear energy created enough of an impetus to rally groups of citizens to recognize the dangers of complete devastation.

Astrophysicist Neil Degrasse Tyson notes that the Environmental Protection Agency was founded in 1970, shortly after we saw the famous earthrise photo of the earth 'rising' over the horizon of the moon. Before that planet-sized selfie was snapped, earth had never been pictorially represented with clouds and atmosphere. That picture prompted a number of people to launch preservation efforts on national and international scales. Tyson also states that there is no 'center' in the universe, for it is constantly expanding in every direction. A central point would be impossible to find in an ever-shifting, transient cosmos.

The mythologist Joseph Campbell had his own take on the earthrise photograph. He viewed it as physical proof that we are not at the center of any system, rather part of a much greater whole. "Is the center the earth? Is the center the moon? The center is anywhere you like… The rising earth shows none of those divisive territorial lines that on our maps are so conspicuous and important. The chosen center may be anywhere. The Holy Land is no special place. It is every place that has ever been recognized and mythologized by any people as home."

In this light violence no longer makes sense. There was once a biological imperative for murder. In small tribes it was kill or be killed. We have evolved tremendously in the 10,000 years since urban centers began developing. This facet of group mentality needs to be left behind if we hope to create a prosperous global culture comprised of various societies. Groupishness as cooperation.

We've had much larger issues to address since the riders on Apollo 8 snapped the earth rising. Yet inane cultural war items under guise of religious freedom persist. When the national media advocates for these issues—abortion, anti-marriage equality measures, and, I can't believe I have to write this, geocentrism, the small movement of people who believe the earth *really is* the center of the universe—we are wasting time when an issue like climate change needs immediate attention.

Humanity's relationship to the natural world was in mind when the concept of *ahimsa* was first developed. Before diving deeper into that part of the story, we must understand just what happens when we become angry, the fateful harbinger of violence. To understand what *ahimsa* implies, we need to explore our animal nature from the inside out.

IT WILL BE USEFUL to make a distinction. While anger potentially leads to violence, this does not make anger something to be avoided.

There are many reasons our ancestors became enraged: to protect a partner, their land or food supply; out of hunger or frustration. In these cases, violence ensued. We can empathize with needing to protect our family and community. It turns out that anger itself has beneficial qualities: it lowers the level of the stress hormone cortisol in our blood.

Due to these findings, neuroscientists no longer view anger as a positive or negative emotion. They consider the motivational direction behind it. Anger is a catalyst for change: you engage with something distressing in order to eliminate it. When considering anger, I often think of *kriyas*, such as Breath of Fire and Kapalbhati, breathing exercises that stir up intense emotions. You can apply such intensity to healing—addressing a problem head-on and solving it—or destruction. Anger is therapeutic if used properly.

It comes down to what we are trying to accomplish. Consider Hungarian psychologist Mihaly Csíkszentmihályi's concept of Flow, in which life is comprised of various emotional terrains. The idea is to understand each terrain without falling victim to any of their pleasures or vices. While Flow is generally attributed to athletes 'in the zone,' it is a psychological state accessible to anybody through proper training.

Csíkszentmihályi determined Flow to be a moment of completely focused motivation, when you utilize all of your emotions and mental energy to engage in a task. No emotion is discarded; it's a matter of harnessing the power of each properly. This, he believes, creates greater satisfaction in life. As he writes, "Happiness...is a condition that must be prepared for, cultivated, and defended privately by each person. People who learn to control inner experience will be able to determine the quality of their lives, which is as close as any of us can come to being happy."

Since happiness is a relative state of being, it should not surprise us that reaching this optimal place requires finesse and dedication. Flow also implies having a container for all of our numerous emotions. Thousands of years before the Hungarian writer penned his classic work, Aristotle realized the application of anger could be beneficial. As he writes, "Anybody can become angry—that is easy, but to be angry with the right person and to the right degree and at the right time and for the right purpose, and in the right way—that is not within everybody's power and is not easy."

Civil rights. Women's rights. Mass kidnappings. Sex slave trafficking. Collective anger sharply focused at a target has the potential for great change. Rage as *Drishti*.

While working on Flow Play, Philip and I found that studying music teaches us how our brains work. We devoted a section to protest music, which uses anger in a constructive manner. Questioning cultural power structures inspires us to reinvent the framework. Presenting our case in song encourages empathy in like-minded citizens frustrated by the society we live within.

Professor of Neurology and Neurosurgery Robert Zatorre's work has shown that angry-sounding music creates physiological changes through increased activity of our sympathetic nervous system. Neuroimaging studies revealed an uptick of action in the amygdala, the almond-shape pair of nuclei that play a primary role in decision-making and emotional reactivity, when listening to music associated with anger.

Neuroscientist Jaak Panksepp realized our abundance of space for thought allows us to incubate schemes for justice when wronged. For example, babies as young as six months old understand fair play. When shown videos of puppets either helping or harming others, they will almost always choose the helpful chap when offered real life versions of the puppets, even going so far as to snub the offenders. A variety of animals recognize fairness as well, including the canine running around in your living room. If you have two dogs, try giving one of them two bones and another only one and see what happens. Cats, while more conspicuous, will quickly make sure you know they have observed an injustice.

For millennia protest songs have roused cultures to fight the power. Tribes used rage-filled chants to frighten invaders; armies blasted angry music to motivate soldiers. English psychiatrist Anthony Storr writes that music serves a primary communal function by binding citizens together, dating back 100,000 years to the fires our ancestors danced around.

Today yoga creates similar communal bonds, sometimes with its own soundtrack. Yet in many classes anger is treated as an aberration. I've never heard an American *kirtan* singer chant mantras in low growls or play their instruments in minor keys. To hear that sort of deep despair I tune in to Indian *bhajans*, where the multifaceted complexity of our emotional world expresses the totality of our experiences.

Singers despair and rage because anger feels satisfying. It excites primitive areas in our brains meant for protection, foraging and self-defense. The time between a triggered event and a response from the amygdala can be as little as a quarter of a second. Almost at the same time blood flow increases to the frontal lobe—specifically the part of the brain just over the left eye, which controls reasoning. The frontal lobes are the rational part of our brain, making sure other regions are kept in check. These lobes keep us from striking out with physical violence, as well as following the direction of least resistance.

We first feel an emotion and then react. Increasing the distance between experiencing the emotion and expressing it through action is part of what yoga and meditation address. The frontal lobes are the main control center for attention. They keep our minds from wandering and focused on the task at hand. It is here that anger is harvested and used as a catalyst for transformation. Yogis learn to remain focused and calm during intense situations by rewiring our brains to surrender in difficult poses. In yoga we also practice not allowing anger to turn into jealousy, hatred or violence. The Warrior postures symbolically represent determined anger, bodily metaphors exhibiting fury as a focal point of change.

At first glance this seems counterintuitive. I attribute this as being a failure of imagination, not a hidden feature of yoga. The lord of yoga, Shiva, is also Natraj, the dancer whose destruction of the universe gives birth to new possibilities. Compartmentalizing emotions leads to labeling, bringing further stress when we wind up in a compartment we didn't intend to walk into. Navigating all of our inner world's twists and turns proves much healthier, as Csíkszentmihályi writes. To become fully human, we have to fully express our range of emotional colors.

We share this penchant for intensity with all mammals. Jaak Panksepp assigns anger to our RAGE system (he capitalizes the brain's seven systems to denote their scientific basis), which runs from the medial areas of the amygdala down the curved pathway of the stria terminalis to the media hypothalamus, on to specific areas of the periacqueductal gray (PAG). This system can be provoked in animals through electrical stimulation. When tested in humans, they clenched their jaws and reported intense anger absent any rational reason for being irritated.

I've listened to people tease apart their mental and emotional worlds, as if the dry logic of their brain, useful for keeping track of finances and arriving at work on time, is in conflict with the rich universe of emotions, that mystical field from on high that defines their 'true' character. This misunderstanding of how our brains operate has caused great confusion and led to tragic consequences. Emotions are as much part of our neural structure as the brain regions allowing you to read these words right now. To wrap our heads around the intricate dance of the passions and rationality we'll soon investigate one of the greatest cases of *himsa* (violence) the world has ever known. First, a little more about how our brains operate.

AHIMSA IS VEIWED AS THE primary component in conquering the emotions and actions causing destruction. This most distinctive aspect of the yoga practice also serves as the foundation of India's major spiritual traditions: Buddhism, Hinduism and Jainism. Patanjali considered *ahimsa* an integral part of the *maha-vrata* (great vow), which must be observed under all circumstances.

The historically important emphasis on non-harming reaches back into our ancient neurobiology from our evolution as mammals. Our ethical principles did not originate with religious traditions. They are nature-based developments from our history as animals with social emotions. Certain branches of science—evolutionary biology, anthropology and neurobiology—have shown that ethical behaviors, including the notion of nonviolence, are a subset of social behaviors shared by many mammals and birds alike. Dutch primatologist and ethologist Frans de Waal writes that numerous animals survive through cooperation and sharing, wolves, killer whales, and primates among them.

It appears our revered prophets of compassion had many wise, fanged, furry, and feathered predecessors. Such altruistic behavior pertains to a group: in non-human animals, non-harming is confined to the pack. Among humans this begins with family, extends to the tribe, and only recently, city or nation. Luckily as a species we lean in an ethical direction, armed as we are with an innate empathy. However, we are also the most superstitious of all creatures. Our religions have strong in-group biases. In a more globalized society the challenge lies in establishing universal non-harming encompassing all sentient creatures, not just 'chosen' humans.

Scientifically speaking, emotions and our neurobiological dispositions have given birth to our moral behavior. The greatest enforcer of compassion is derived from our animal emotions. De Waal offers vivid examples of emotionally guided moral behavior in non-human animals: elephants recruiting friends to help pull a heavy box, chimps refusing undeserved rewards, bonobos comforting losers after a fight.

Over the last few decades, neuroscientific studies have shown the ways in which emotions affect human beings' moral and social behavior. For example, when healthy individuals sustain brain damage to regions necessary for processing certain emotions and feelings, their ability to live normal lives is drastically altered. The social arena is an area of particular difficulty for people whose emotions are blunted. The evolutionary reasons for empathy, compassion, forgiveness, gratitude, mindfulness, reverence for life and trust become apparent. These qualities help make society work better for everyone, as well making *ahimsa* such a constructive force.

Countless neurotransmitters help us survive by making us feel a particular way (warm and fuzzy), consequently associating the feeling with the action causing it. Chemicals act on neurons to produce desired results. An adolescent male brain awash with testosterone becomes violent and hyper-sexed; a body overloaded with endorphins will set off our fight/flight/freeze reflex. Endogenous opioids and oxytocin play a huge role in all social emotions.

Over the last few decades, researchers from varied disciplines of neuroscience have realized nonviolence has another important component with the discovery of mirror neurons. These neurons are a subset of the motor neurons that activate when we move our leg or when someone touches our arm. They not only fire when something touches our body, but also when we see *someone else's body* being touched. These neurons turn on in exactly the same way in each situation. This is what makes us feel squeamish when we see violence done to others (or in movies) and physically 'feel' their pain. Importantly, this is what makes us refrain from harming others.

In a certain way, your neurons are acting as though what you see around you is happening *to you*. Neuroscientist and neurobiologist Antonio Damasio calls this effect the 'as-if-body-loop.' The brain uses incoming body signals like clay to sculpt a particular body state based on a false construction, not a real body state. This is the physical underpinning of empathy and feeling connected to others, affording this aspect of neuroscience with major implications for learning more about how we might create a worldview governed by nonviolence—and not only to other human beings.

AHIMSA WAS INITIALLY DEVELOPED to ponder the relationship between humans and animals, not humans and other humans. Animal sacrifices were a regular feature of rituals. The bond between culture and cosmos depended on the gods getting a carnivorous fix. As city-states evolved and citizens observed the seemingly limitless power of priests, the necessity of this rite was called into question. Yet people still wanted their meat. Guilt may have well produced the first use of the term, not as an act of passivity, instead as a double negative: I will do no harm, even though the animal will be slaughtered. Entire lists were developed over the centuries regarding the proper means of killing animals, and not just in India.

Other cultures assume this psychology. I sometimes hear the word 'intention' in association with meat consumption. Saying a prayer before dinner is believed to magically absolve the eater of bad karma associated with the murder necessary in producing the meat. This has nothing to do with the animal; it alleviates the culpability of the human consumer. This prayer ignores the biological drive of every life form: preservation of species. *Ahimsa* may very well be rooted in such a perplexing mindset.

As Indian scholar Wendy Doniger writes, this problem far exceeds the capacity of the individual: "Nonviolence became a cultural idea for Hindus precisely because it holds out the last hope of a cure, all the more desirable since unattainable, for a civilization that has, like most, always suffered from chronic and terminal violence."

America is no different. A trail of tears follows our every step, from the bloody founding of this country to the violence necessary for creating the wide economic rift currently dominating our social structure. Billionaires treat our working class like *Shudra*, an integral part of the modern social fabric. There are many ways to be violent. Not all of them involve physical pain.

Disregarding others is a persistent feature of societies. It is not surprising that we treat other species with no regard at all.

Humans have long applied Skinner's theory of behaviorism—animals are merely programmed, robotic creatures with no original thoughts—to the entirety of the animal kingdom. Biomedical and pharmacological testing, as well as meat and fur production, flourished during the reign of behaviorism. While it took psychologists, with the help of neuroscientists, decades to undo the damage of Skinner's ideology, we remain far behind in comprehending just how advanced the brains of other creatures really are. If we did understand how closely related they are to us, we might tune down the violence quite a bit.

For over 150 years rats have been used in laboratory experiments. Roughly 95% of all animals tested are rodents. They share many genetic, biological and behavioral characteristics with humans, making them ideal candidates for the job. Still we assume that rats do not feel emotions or understand the pain associated with experimentation. Jaak Panksepp has proved otherwise.

Using a handheld bat detector—bat signals are 120 to 160 kilohertz to rats' fifty kilohertz; humans hear at two-four kilohertz—Panksepp realized rats laugh while being tickled. Once you flip them over and rub your fingers lightly over their bellies, the furry creatures seek out your hand, provided you haven't pet your cat that morning. Then they will run away, even if they've never encountered a feline before.

Scientists are wary of anthropomorphizing animals. It's easy to assign human characteristics to the smiling dog or playful dolphin. Dolphins and humans began diverging 100 million years ago, so the notion of us sharing social habits seems preposterous. Yet a big part of our problem when contemplating the animal kingdom is just how much we've removed ourselves from it. Religions have pounded it into our heads that we are a separate being entirely, all those woolly and scaly creatures 'put' here for our usage however we see fit.

This is obviously not the case. Take play, which a sizable proportion of animals engage in. Panksepp found play rooted in the brain's PLAY system. It is an important component of social bonding. Trust is developed through it. Watch two dogs wrestle and you might at first grow alarmed at their fierce fangs. Unless the tumble turns violent, blood never flows. This style of nipping is exhibited in cats, dolphins, and rats as well. Soccer players and boxers have even tried it out. Play keeps us cognizant of boundaries while offering an outlet for creative expression. Contrary to the lingering delusion of behaviorism, it is an *emotional* behavior. We need play.

"The emotional mind is the *most* visible part of an animal's brain," Panksepp says. "You can see it directly by watching the animal's behavior, and you can hear it in their vocalizations."

Play also triggers the release of proteins that help build regions such as the amygdala, hippocampus, and prefrontal cortex, where we make decisions. Turns out tumbling down the hill and playing hide-and-seek provide irreplaceable educational training.

Not only do other animals share our capacity for emotional expression, but as it turns out, for cognition as well. Bowerbirds are artists, arranging their nests in aesthetically pleasing diagrams using found objects to attract females. Rats also partake in metacognition: they know what they know and make informed decisions. They dream just as we do. Elephants, whales, and great apes share with us von Economo cells, spindle-shaped neurons that aid in developing empathy, emotional suffering, love and sociality.

One of the most abused species on our planet, chickens, turns out to be highly intelligent. Special microphones picked up twenty-four different vocalizations signaling a variety of needs and fears. These birds share with dolphins a wily and vicious side, going to lengths to expose other males to danger or deny them the luxury of lying with the ladies. The automatic behaviors Skinner had suggested are actually the result of numerous cognitive traits.

As Carolynn L. Smith and Sarah L. Zielinski write in *Scientific American* about these studies, "The findings also have ethical implications for how society treats farmed chickens: recognizing that chickens have these cognitive traits compels moral considerations of the conditions they endure as a result of production systems designed to make chicken meat and eggs as widely available and cheap as possible."

Over ten billion animals are killed every year for food in the United States. (I've seen global totals range from fifty-eight to eighty billion.) Our national population was 313.9 million as of 2012, accounting for nearly thirty-two animals per American. When meat arrives shrink wrapped in Whole Foods, it's easy to deny an emotional animal not all that different from us—dreaming, caring for its family, not immune to suffering, aware of the world around it—provided the protein. Just because animals cannot communicate in English does not imply they cannot speak at all. We are only now learning their many languages.

While we should take caution in personifying other species, we must not separate ourselves too far from their livelihood and suffering, as it has and will continue to affect our own. Climate change has been in part attributed to increased toxicity in factory farming. A recent UN report revealed that as global warming persists, societies are likely to become more violent again, a trend that will counteract Pinker's research cited above. With depleting animal sources, not to mention water—I write this during California's worst drought in recorded history—our overuse of resources is rapidly changing our society for the worse. Animal protein might have once been required for our ancestors, but those days have passed given our increased knowledge of nutritional science. The 'need' for meat is another archaic remnant.

Ahimsa was dreamed up in part to address one specific regional issue: we love eating cows, but we love the ghee they provide more. How to save the species to get what we really want? The problem was a social one. Vegetarianism in India was implemented for food rationing and, later, to deny invading Muslim tribes the right to slaughter the cows needed for dairy. The spiritual nature was added later as a romanticized justification. Today we face our own dilemma: knowing that animals share a wide range of cognitive and emotional traits with us, can we in good heart continue to slaughter them by the billions, especially when the destruction of their ecosystems is eroding our own?

Individuals in a society unite to address the tribulations of their day. Sometimes one person rises above the chatter to help forge a new understanding of what's really going on around. Martin Luther King, Jr. was one such man, and it is to him we return to conclude this chapter.

AS HE SAT IN BLUMSTEIN'S Department Store in Harlem signing copies of his new book, *Strive Toward Freedom*, King was approached by an African-American woman. Izola Ware Curry asked if he was indeed the famous author. He replied yes. She revealed a letter opener, driving it deep into his chest.

It took a number of hours for the doctors at Harlem Hospital to remove the blade. It had been pressing directly against his aorta. If King had sneezed the large artery would have ruptured, bleeding him to death in minutes. His life was spared by millimeters.

While in the hospital, King issued a statement on September 30, 1958, just ten days after the stabbing: "The pathetic aspect of this experience is not the injury to one individual. It demonstrates that a climate of hatred and bitterness so permeates areas of our nation that inevitably deeds of extreme violence must erupt. Today, it was I. Tomorrow it could be anther leader or any man, woman or child who will be the victim of lawlessness and brutality. I hope this experience proves to be socially constructive by demonstrating the urgent necessity for nonviolence to govern the affairs of men."

At a time when someone had committed the most violent act possible against any one person, King devoted himself more fully to the application of nonviolence. He decided nothing was in the way of his visiting India. Just four months after being released, King traveled around Gandhi's homeland with his wife, Coretta, and confidante Lawrence Reddick for five weeks. Americans might never have heard the 'I Have a Dream' speech if not for this man's refusal to submit to bitterness.

The violence we do to ourselves: thoughts of insufficiency and despair; the way we look; what we don't own; where we're not at. The violence to other humans: judgment; gossip; Internet trolling; religious bigotry; beating partners, useless wars, senseless killings. That we commit against other species: animals confined in pens so small they cannot turn around, kept alive on pharmaceuticals in order to feed us the most tender cut; fooling ourselves with terms like 'conscious consumerism' and 'free range,' pretending family farmers make murder enjoyable; the hipster cults of bone luges and foie gras. Life may feed on life and all life may be suffering, but that does not mean we have to add fuel to the fire when other options exist.

Nonviolence requires practice and patience. It does not come easy. But together we can achieve it, if we so choose.

To pick out threads of violence is to unweave an ancient carpet that is as much a part of our birthright as any other survival mechanism. Knowing this, do we persist by consciously partaking in the violent acts we commit? Diligence and perseverance are required. We don't have to be a King to set into motion the changes we wish to see, but we do need to accept the violence we commit while taking steps to correct it.

Buddhism reveals its yogic roots in its concept of the bodhisattva vow: no one is liberated until we all are. We've put one foot forward in considering the most prominent: violence. There are nine more steps to take.

2 ASTEYA : GIVE IT AWAY NOW

SHEILA RAMOS HAS NOT lived a particularly unusual life. The Hawaii native married at seventeen; by nineteen she was through with her husband. She took her two small children and moved to Alaska to begin anew. Now fifty-eight, having spent decades in Alaska and Florida, the grandmother once again lives in her home state on a patch of rural land. Only now the roof over her head is made of tarp, not wood and tile.

Ramos is a working woman. The cosmetology degree she earned shortly after leaving Hawaii led to various salon jobs, eventually landing her a gig selling cosmetics at J.C. Penney. That turned into a management position, where she rocked business suits all day. Eventually, however, she wanted to work with her hands, so she took a cue from her longtime partner, an electrician who ran a side business mixing and pouring concrete. Ramos started a small construction company, successful for years until another company outbid her and forced her to close shop.

By that time Ramos was done with Alaskan temperatures, moving with her eighty-three-year-old mother and three grandchildren—she won custody after one of her children was arrested on drug-related charges—to Florida. Selling her parents' home in Hawaii, she was able to buy a $300,000 home with no mortgage or debt. A serial entrepreneur, she took out a $90,000 mortgage on her house in 2004 to start her own lawn-care business. Within a few months she had forty customers, easily paying off the $790 monthly payment.

The following year a New Jersey driver visiting Florida cut her off, causing Ramos to crash. Her injuries forced her to stop working. Within six months she could no longer pay off that mortgage. She took out another for $140,000, upping her monthly payment to $1,150, which she paid off in part with credit cards. Another $28,000 against her house helped her son buy a trailer but did nothing to help her own situation. Refinancing again the following year, the $262,000 mortgage against her $403,000 house should have left her in the clear, even though her monthly payment was now up to $2,200. Unfortunately she didn't know her agent had written down her monthly income as $6,500. He was only over her house for fifteen minutes; she never read through the entire document.

Ramos, of course, was not alone in such thinking. During the period from 2004-2006, American homeowners borrowed nearly $1.5 trillion against their homes. Such a startling national economic boost could never sustain. When Ramos returned to Hawaii to live on a small piece of land her family still owned, it would not be in a house. Today she survives in a tent, her grandchildren wondering where the roof went.

AMERICA HAS FEW RITUALS. As comedian Joe Rogan commented on one of his podcasts, you turn eighteen and then what are you supposed to do? The traditional path leads to a job, or college and then a job, or graduate school to job, and so on. As an old friend once said, 'You work at work until work works on you.' Everything relies on an employment model that is no longer relevant to a growing portion of the population. Outside of a job, little exists to ensure the symbolic passage to adulthood: no wrestling a lion, no full back tattoo, no sitting alone in a tent for a week in complete isolation. Perhaps we've forgotten a few things about being human that 'primitives' understood.

Owning a house has long been married to the job ethos. This is by design. In 1919 the U.S. government helped re-launch the Own Your Own Home campaign. An ambitious Secretary of Commerce, Herbert Hoover, announced, "maintaining a high percentage of individual homeowners is one of the searching tests that now challenge the people of the United States." Nine years later President Hoover signed into law economic stimulus initiatives to help Americans buy homes, which initially teetered along due to the Great Depression. No matter, homeownership remained a governmental goal. In the following decades the suburbs helped solidify a house's special place in the social imagination.

In more recent times, presidents Bill Clinton and George W. Bush aimed for a combined 13.5 million new homeowners during their tenures. This fascination with ownership feeds everyone: for the homeowner, a place to call their own, plant a garden, raise a family, modify to their whims, as well as a sense of rooting; to the government, it gives form to a nation, fitting neatly into the 'Make Your Dreams Come True' ethos this country clings to; to banks, mortgages are gold, plain and simple. In this fantasy, everyone wins.

Until everybody loses.

It would be easy to write a chapter on *asteya*, non-stealing, by investigating the banks, which nearly brought down the global economy by selling an endless stream of toxic mortgages, or the government that enabled them to do so through a total lack of regulations. Both these entities played a major role in destroying an integral aspect of the imagined American dream; both were thieves in their own ways.

But this book is about what *we* can do. Perhaps some citizens should have known better than signing a mortgage after putting down next to nothing. Look no further than Sheila Ramos. She should have been more cautious with her agent. Yet her story, like those of so many others, is nuanced. The catalyst for her economic downturn was not overspending, but an injury that she was never properly compensated for.

There's something deeper at play here, however, dealing with our perception of money and the value of objects, a beneficial lesson in how we steal from ourselves due to an unhealthy relationship to fantasies. To better understand that lesson, we need to gaze back at yoga's role in America over the last 121 years, for it offers a powerful insight into how we think and act.

WHEN SWAMI VIVEKANANDA introduced yoga philosophy to the Parliament of World Religions in Chicago in 1893, Americans were taken by his eloquence and charm, as well as his ideas of unification among the planet's faiths. Instead of preaching a fundamentalist insistence of one story being true for everyone, his open-mindedness was a breath of fresh air, a calming round of emotional *pranayama* for the crowds when he spoke lines such as, "A story is a flame that burns no less brightly if strangers light their candles from it."

His Hinduism was syncretic, as much of Hinduism has proven to be over the millennia. He welcomed other prophets and leaders, exploring their ideas as woven into the rich tapestry of his own tradition. While his feelings on science were questionable—he believed that people being born happy or sad was due to past incarnations, not genetics and social conditions—his wit and knowledge were infectious, his persona playing a large role in carving an early niche for yoga philosophy in this country.

Not that yoga was new. Ralph Waldo Emerson had already helped publish a translation of the *Bhagavad Gitā* over a half-century earlier, taking a cue from his father, William, the first American to translate a Sanskrit text in 1805. Theosophist Helena Blavatsky crafted her own multicultural secret society, including yoga texts, decades before Vivekananda's arrival.

Truth be told, the swami's influence after the conference would be brief. His legacy only became widespread in recent years. Even with a name translating as 'bliss master,' for well over a half-century after his visit many Americans viewed yoga with a suspicious eye.

During the first decade of the twentieth century over one million immigrants poured into the country each year, setting off a rampant backlash by families of former immigrants who felt the land now belonged to them. Fashion and cuisine arriving from the 'exotic' East might be acceptable, but the actual people and their philosophies, languages and cultural mores, were another story.

Around the same time Hoover was cheerleading for homeowners Congress overwhelmingly passed the Immigration Act of 1917, not-so-affectionately known as the Asiatic Barred Zone Act. The law excluded homosexuals, anarchists, alcoholics, idiots—not sure how that's defined, but it was in there—and feeble-minded persons, as well as, just to drive the point home, anyone from China or India, from entering the country. It took nearly three decades to repeal.

You can imagine how well yoga went over. The press went to town on the 'Hindu love cults' popping up on the West coast, later in upstate New York and eventually Manhattan. One of the early proponents was Perry Baker, who at age thirteen befriended a Tantric yogi in Iowa. Baker studied at this guru's feet for a decade, eventually reintroducing himself to the public as Pierre Arnold Bernard, the first American yogi.

Bernard was different than most swamis flying over from India looking for American clientele. He focused on meditation and breathing techniques in order to enter alternate states of consciousness; he too was a bliss master. Only Bernard emphasized postures for physical vitality and health, something many Indians thought to be lowly and unnecessary for attaining elevated states of consciousness. Vivekananda for one spoke against the fascination with headstands, backbends and so on.

At the same time Bernard started teaching *asanas*—freely adjusting his female practitioners, a habit landing him in trouble with the law on more than one occasion—a burgeoning nationalism in

India was inspiring yogis to combine wrestling, weightlifting, and gymnastics as a response to nearly two centuries of British rule. Today the Warrior series is more the result of fed-up Indian nationalists ready to strike down an oppressive government than blissing out in Tantric rituals.

The battle of yoga was in full swing by the 1920's, when Bernard relocated to Nyack, New York, bankrolled by starry-eyed members of the Vanderbilt family, whose fortune helped fuel his latest venture in yoga combined with circus acts, vaudeville and, oddly, baseball. To say the man lived an eccentric life would be an understatement.

While Bernard was getting everyone fit, a charismatic swami named Yogananda was telling Americans they use their body too much. He claimed a little will power is all that is needed. It worked. His own will led his followers to purchase a hilltop retreat in Malibu for his Self-Realization Fellowship—land he almost lost due to accusations of property fraud.

Slowly America's broad disdain of yoga and things associated with it—at the time, astral projection, telekinesis, clairvoyance, and, if you've ever read *Autobiography of a Yogi*, claims of animated dead bodies—was loosening as the handsome nephew of Pierre Bernard, Theos, returned to America after supposedly being venerated as the 'first White Lama' in Tibet. He was later killed there, but not before his stealthy physique was pinned on many walls, inspiring a wave of yogic fitness still going strong today.

Not that everything went smoothly for this Indian craft. When Eleanor Roosevelt was accused of practicing yoga in the White House, she claimed that she didn't know her daily headstand was considered a yogic exercise. Communism was the fear word of the day: Indian prime minister Nehru promised Americans that he was not secretly training Russian cosmonauts to breathe better in space.

Shortly after these events yoga, the physical practice, was being taught in YMCA's across America. The floodgates loosened. Renowned violinist Yehudi Menuhin sang yoga's virtues thanks to his friendship with B.K.S. Iyengar, who helped him sleep one day after dealing with tour insomnia. Menuhin carted Iyengar around the world to teach small groups of friends, helping the yogi achieve international fame and respect.

And then, of course, there was the Beatles. Countless Americans swear by the Transcendental Meditation techniques as espoused by their beloved, then scorned, Maharishi Mahesh Yogi. Yoga might have been part of the counterculture, but the counterculture had infiltrated the mainstream. The discipline might not yet have had the broad reach it does today, but it was certainly no longer seen as a foreign threat. Yoga as a stress relieving, muscle-toning regimen was here to stay. Yet something odd happened on the way to the multi-billion dollar business that is yoga in 2014. It was introduced to Samuel Smiles.

WELL BEFORE THE KINDLE AND IPAD, nearly a century-and-a-half prior to the explosion of print-on-demand titles, Samuel Smiles was in a bind. The Scottish author's book, *Self-Help: with Illustrations of Character and Conduct*, was rejected by Routledge in 1855. Another publisher, John Murray, offered to publish it on a half profits system. Smiles felt too invested in the work and wouldn't allow concessions. The government reformer was an entrepreneur. He self-published the work.

Smiles sold 20,000 copies in the first year, a hefty sum for the lone investor. When the man passed forty-nine years later, *Self-Help* had sold over a quarter-million copies. He was lauded as an inspired guru, publishing other works such as *Character*, *Thrift*, and *Duty*, though none did as well as his initial foray into literature. Smiles enjoyed immense fame while alive. Little could he have known an entire genre would be created from his insightful book.

While somewhat tame by today's standards, *Self*-Help includes expectable jargon, though Smiles himself was a devotee of failure: he heralded its virtue at every turn, reminding readers that failure, not success, teaches life's greatest lessons. In this he was in good company: inventors like Thomas Edison and Benjamin Franklin also cherished missteps, even if they are remembered for what they did in fact accomplish. They knew those achievements were impossible without thousands of blunders along the way.

Which is why it was odd watching Smiles' genre become co-opted, predominantly in the nineties and especially over the last decade, by a new wave of self-help authors rebranding his messages while removing the lingo of failure. These writers represent a new way of approaching life: success is ultimately (and always) guaranteed, fumbles along the way only a lesser version of the destined you. With Smiles, failure was a beautiful part of the process; in fact, he valued the *process* over the goal. Not so our positive psychology coaches offering everything imaginable in six steps, eight rules and ten universal maxims.

Let me make clear an important point: I am not saying to not think positively. Positivity is an essential component of a healthy mental and emotional life. As I write this I'm currently going through cancer. Upon learning of my illness a close friend, a doctor in Atlanta, told me 70% of my healing would be in my attitude. While I cannot quantify any such number, I fully agreed. My recovery has been educational, emotionally enriching and, even with its challenges, rewarding. I attribute this to staying positive throughout the entire experience, even when fears and sadness almost got the best of me.

The positive psychology mentality I'm discussing is more sinister. It states that *everything* is going to be all right, every time. If it's not, it must be the fault of the universe, another way of saying *I* was doing something wrong to deserve this—an unfortunate relic of karma as espoused by Vivekananda and others, that we are the product of past failures. This way of thinking piles on guilt: every misstep is either the result of misguided action or part of a 'plan' that will ultimately resolve itself. If it never does, that's part of the plan, too, and something *better* is waiting still. In the promise of better we make choices that do not serve us, which, as we will see, figured heavily into the recent housing crash.

The tragedy occurs when we find ourselves waiting instead of failing. Worse, we don't accept responsibility for our failures because it's only another step to something bigger, regardless of who gets harmed in the process. By not failing we're not learning. We shrink. The ultimate robbery of the last decade didn't come at the hands of the banks or the government. We stole from ourselves.

LIKE MANY THINGS INDIAN, *asteya*, or non-stealing, is to be understood symbolically and literally. The basic gist is easy enough: if it's not yours, don't take it. The *Yoga Bhashya* goes a step further, asking the yogi to abstain from appropriating things belonging to another without permission. The *Shandilya Upanishad* suggests not coveting another's property, mentally, vocally or physically. *Asteya* always implied not messing with people's heads.

Yet yogis messing with heads have been constant. I'm not referring to the mental and emotional reorganization when adhering to the principles of yoga, or any of the attempts of reaching the so-called higher states of consciousness, such as Gopi Krishna's popular account of Kundalini. I mean the human weaknesses too often coinciding with power: the elevated status of the teacher, or as history has termed him, the guru.

To this day commentary about the necessity of the guru persists. It is believed to honor the traditional blueprint of yoga: you find a teacher, study with him—women practicing yoga is a recent phenomenon—treat his every word as law. Eventually, if you pay close enough attention and dedicate yourself fully, you might one day become a teacher yourself. This apprenticeship model makes sense if you and your teacher end up on equal footing. As you can imagine, and as we have seen over and over, the failings of this framework are abundant.

Chandra Mohan Jain is a case in point. The Kuchwada native spent his entire life attempting to overcome stigmas attached with a small village upbringing. Renaming himself Acharya Rajneesh a few years after his supposed enlightenment at age twenty-one in 1953, the university lecturer became known as a dynamic and intelligent speaker, a trait leading to trouble with the Indian government. Besides his suspect take on Tantric philosophy—he became known as the 'sex guru'—Rajneesh railed against Gandhi, who he bitterly criticized for celebrating poverty. The idea of purposefully living in squalor would prove antithetical to Rajneesh's entire philosophical system.

Today you'll find Osho quotes plastered across yoga studios and on social media all over the world, but during his American life he was known as Bhagwan Shree Rajneesh, yet another incarnation assumed before moving to Oregon in 1981. He had already taken advantage of the Americans visiting his Pune ashram and decided to move to his source of wealth. In short order he acquired an entire fleet of Rolls Royce's, preaching the prosperity gospel at every turn. His followers worshipped his every word, yet the structure of the guru dissolved: there would be no one beyond Rajneesh; he was the ultimate purveyor of spiritual knowledge. Let the Gandhians spin their loincloths, Osho had expensive cars to be chauffeured around in. Ninety-three in total.

Rajneesh's American vacation was short-lived. Four years later he was deported, effectively running from bioterrorism and attempted murder charges. His followers had planned to poison the food supply of the surrounding region, the Dalles, as well as attempted to assassinate a local politician (as well as kill each other). Rajneesh's early love of socialism had given way to a fond appreciation for capitalism. The locals who were giving him problems regarding his compound would have to be strong-armed out or killed. He also ran into trouble for not paying property taxes.

Osho was the name he assumed near the end of his life, shortly after twenty-one countries denied him entry. Today you'll find his many books, lectures, calendars, and tarot card decks front and center in New Age bookshops and yoga studios, a testament to the man who wanted to stick it to the man. Free sex, a love of profit this prophet would never be ashamed of, the rebel to inspire liberal rebellions: Osho was the ideal counterrevolutionary whose life few would ever literally follow. So much easier it is to post two sentences from one of his talks than investigate his actual life.

Still, it is those talks surviving, not his reported addiction to nitric oxide and Valium; not his advice to euthanize children born deaf, dumb or blind; not his feelings that gas chambers quickly brought Jews to God; not his announcement that homosexuals created AIDS and had fallen from human dignity; not his followers' engineering of mass poisoning, attempted murder, or land takeover, nor his badmouthing all-things American when returning to India in 1985. Osho died at age fifty-eight of heart failure, sending his followers on witch hunts for the person supposedly sickening him with black magic. His yoga of rebellion and abundance is what loyalists cherish about the man today, even if his actual life was antithetical to pretty much every ethical code in this book.

The gurus who have appeared in America mostly arrive with carefully tailored messages designed to appeal to American sensibilities. Never would the asceticism of meditation and breathing techniques attract legions of liberal middle- and upper-class followers, the crowd needed to support their travels and exceedingly lavish lifestyles. Besides, claiming to have risen above materialism is a fantastic way to acquire objects, as well as have sex with pretty young acolytes.

The rigors of yoga philosophy and practice have been compromised in focusing on the results, a pattern Patanjali explicitly warned against. But we want the glory without the suffering. Because of this yoga became a bedfellow with the positive psychology movement: you were born to inherit whatever you want, so take it in all your God-given glory. Just don't forget to pay the messenger.

Joel and Diana Kramer, authors of the influential *The Guru Papers: Masks of Authoritarian Power*, are experts in the deception propagated by gurus. These men (and increasingly women) are masters of observing character traits in would-be followers. One of the most important qualities is self-trust. Without it, the Kramer's write, people are "subject to easy manipulation."

This trend is not limited to Indian swamis. The prosperity theology of American televangelist Creflo Dollar is a perfect example. He preaches that God rewards faith, not to mention donations to the church. In 2006 alone, Dollar's congregation of over 30,000 members kicked in $69 million. Prosperity is certainly working for the man: two Rolls Royce's—a paltry sum compared to ninety-three, but still—a private jet and multiple multi-million dollar homes keep Dollar singing the dollar's praises.

The country's largest televangelist, Joel Osteen, isn't called the 'smiling preacher' for nothing. He purposefully avoids the hard lessons, choosing to focus on the fruits. He recognized early on that church was no place for heavy discussions on theology. Keep it focused on what his followers can achieve, not what they have to sacrifice, a fitting parallel to the gurus of last century. Worth a reported $56.5 million, one of Osteen's beloved lectures included telling his faithful followers they should not be afraid of dreaming about owning a big house. God would provide the capital from somewhere, somehow. Unfortunately for them, and for America, they listened.

AMERICA TURNED THE CORNER of the new millennium in great shape. The first dot-com bubble hadn't burst. Our president played saxophone; he didn't come from an elitist crowd, he had to fight his way there—the perpetual fable of the underachiever done good. Disposable income seemed everywhere, even if really it wasn't. When Bush charged ahead into multiple wars, the public went on a spending spree. Remember his post-9/11 advice that we should shop to lift America out of the doldrums? Nationalism perfectly merged with capitalism. You couldn't beat the opportunity: banks offered such great deals on homes few could resist. Besides, it was our American birthright. We'd been working hard on achieving this goal for over eighty years. Damn if a little thing like money was going to get in the way of our manifest destiny.

The culture of positive thinking is not the culture of critical thinking, however. In this, we've suffered tremendously. If reality curves toward happiness and abundance, why do we even bother trying to stay positive? Shouldn't it already just be ours? Or could this incessant focus on things always being better—every misstep a 'lesson,' every failure planted by some omnipotent trickster—cover up something much more disturbing in our psyche? Journalist Barbara Ehrenreich tackled this very subject: "Positive thinking may be a quintessentially American activity, associated in our minds with both individual and national success, but it is driven by a terrible insecurity."

These are the same insecurities gurus and prosperity preachers have been exploiting for centuries: we're not good enough, not rich enough, not pretty enough, not *whole*. Perhaps it's because they too do not feel complete, or maybe they recognize a good business opportunity when they see one. They might begin with good intentions and get caught up in the extravagance of wealth as their fan base grows, taunted by and then addicted to the seductive power of tens of thousands of adoring eyes waiting for you to tell them what they want to hear. And you have to tell them that, for if you didn't, they'll find someone who will.

In the slow transformation from the basics necessary for survival to the culture of excess, America's hunger continues to increase. More can only lead to more because what we already have is never quite enough. We don't even notice the tragedy of our comedy: in order to survive our culture, like our body, needs to be in a state of homeostasis. Abundance in any regard is never a good thing. When we fill our brains with ambitions of more—more happiness, more love, more fulfillment, more house—we'll never feel sated. What's been stolen is our integrity, our sense of humanity, and by subscribing to the belief that we aren't already enough, I'm not even sure we can call it stealing. We gave it all away.

3 SAUCHA : CLEANING UP

BLUFFTON, INDIANA IS KNOWN AS the 'Parlor City.' Over a century ago newly paved streets inspired residents to claim that the city was as clean as a parlor. The nickname stuck.

On April 17, 2012, Chandler Gerber set off on one of those sanitized roads to his job cleaning tar pits. En route the twenty-two-year-old traded text messages with his wife, mostly about their newborn daughter. As he drove east on 124—in the direction of Decatur, of Ohio—Gerber switched his attention between his phone and the sun, rapidly gaining potency at five to eight in the morning.

Gerber would have noticed the sights, had he been paying attention: Fair View Cemetery, Elm Grove Cemetery, the landscape of farms and fields unfolding once you roll past Johns Creek. Maybe he would also have seen the Amish wagon carrying a family that has sworn off technology and other modern conveniences in lieu of a pastoral existence.

"This couldn't have happened to me, that couldn't be real. I had to just have dreamed that," Gerber would later say. As he looked down at his phone, three words appeared: I. Love. You.

The next thing he knew a body was rolling from the top of his white GMC van. A few more slumped in the ditch against the barren field. Soon seed would be spread all over these acres, but for now the cemeteries he had just whizzed by provides enough context.

Gerber's van ended up 430 feet from the point of impact. The grill was punched in, the windshield cracked as if a rock or bullet had punctured its surface. As he slowly crept out from the van an older woman, knees bent and head slouched, crouched motionless in the ditch, as if she had just been seated. She had.

Fortunately Mary survived. Not so three of her children. Three-year-old Enos died immediately. Five-year-old Barbara made it all the way to the Fort Wayne emergency room before breathing her last. Seventeen-year-old Jerry, who had been driving the buggy, made it to the hospital before passing on.

And the horse. That's one thing Gerber remembers. Bleeding profusely, body mangled, as confused to his surroundings as the driver who had just slammed into it. Hours later the horse had to be put down as well.

A couple of weeks after the accident, Gerber received a letter from Martin Schwartz, the father of those deceased children. He wrote, "I always wonder if we take enough time with our children. Wishing you the best with your little one in the unknown future. I think of you often. Keep looking up; God is always there. Sincerely, Martin and Mary Schwartz."

Gerber and his family visited the Schwartz's at their invite. They expected, perhaps craved, a short trip. Instead they were there for hours. The people outside of his car were real, just as he and his wife and daughter were living flesh and bone. He would continue to berate himself for spending time focusing on his phone for weeks, for months. Today Gerber travels around the country advocating for the lesson he learned the hard way.

"I wish so bad I could go back to that day and change my focus," Gerber says. "I can do these texts when I get to the stop—there's just nothing that important. *I can text and drive, it's no big deal.* It *is* a big deal. It's life. You get one chance and you live with the choices you make."

SAUCHA MEANS 'PURITY' OR 'CLEANSING.' This technique has always encompassed internal and external cleaning. Inner purity was achieved through clearing out the blemishes of the mind, while the external practice involved water and food. How you took care of yourself inside reflected who you were outside, and vice-versa.

One day I questioned friends online what their daily practice of *saucha* entailed. Everyone mentioned external surroundings or skin: showering daily, doing laundry, eating healthy food, keeping an area of their home clean for meditation. A few remarked about the intertwining of their mental state with their state of cleanliness.

I agreed with all of these. As I exercise and teach daily, I'm constantly showering. My laundry bin never seems to be empty, though I'm at the machines for two to three loads a week. With two cats scurrying around my apartment, the vacuum is in constant demand. My mother used to wake up hours before dawn to clean the house, even though I don't believe it ever got dirty in the first place. While I'm not that ambitious, plenty of her household ethics rubbed off on me. The only space I allow to become cluttered is my desk, which, as a longtime journalist, is par for that particular course. Besides, as Einstein remarked, if cluttered desks reflect cluttered minds, what do empty desks reflect?

When contemplating this *niyama*, however, the idea of writing a chapter on cleaning techniques frightened me. In trainings I've reminded future teachers that appearance is important. Setting an example encompasses many dimensions. I've seen instructors show up just having rolled out of bed still wearing the sweats they slept in. I remember one walking into the studio in jeans and a button down shirt. These are rare albeit scary examples. I didn't think anyone would want to read a chapter on personal hygiene, nor could I be the one to write it.

Instead I'll hone in on inner purity, the ability to fine-tune consciousness to a point of focused attention. Attention and purity might not seem directly related, but in order to achieve a state of mind in alignment with *saucha*, presence of mind is of utmost importance. It made sense to investigate our era's greatest deterrent to accomplishing such a goal: technology.

I'm no technophobe. I won't bother listing all the devices within arm's reach. I build websites, am proficient in graphic design and digital photography, have worked in social media for years. And for years I've struggled with the balance of using technology without becoming used by it. Yes, the latter is a possibility, one that is rapidly altering our very ability to think in the first place. By extension, this trend is affecting our capacity to care for one another in a tragic way.

Texting and driving is not the only manner in which our distractions are getting the best of us. It is an important one, however. Chandler Gerber's story is one of the 100,000 accidents caused by texting drivers each year. At last count, 400,000 people are injured or killed because of distracted driving every year: texting, talking on the phone, and so on. Texting while behind the wheel of a two-ton machine is a deadly habit.

After moving to Los Angeles in 2011 I assumed I'd share the road with good drivers, considering this city was built around the automobile. A devoted subway rider for twelve years, I was amazed at how unprepared drivers are in paying attention to what's going on right in front of them. Checking their phone at a red light is bad enough; whizzing by a texting driver at eighty mph on the 405 is quite literally insane. Yet it happens all the time.

Just as the documentary Gerber is featured in—Warner Herzog's 'From One Second to the Next,' which you can watch on YouTube—I'm sure every driver that causes an accident while texting repeats his sentiment: *I thought I could do it.* Turns out none of us can, and the implications go far deeper than what happens on the highway.

NICHOLAS CARR HAD A PROBLEM. The technology and culture writer penned columns and articles for an impressive list of publications: the *Guardian*, *NY Times*, *Atlantic*, *Wall Street Journal*. His first two books, *Does IT Matter* and *Rewiring the World*, were translated into twenty-five languages. An avid reader and lover of literature, he suddenly found himself unable to finish an entire book.

The writer wasn't alone. He was amazed to learn friends and colleagues were experiencing similar difficulty focusing on long pieces of text. Staring at words on the screen had become torturous, a trend that bled into the printed world. Shortly after starting a blog, he realized reading a book had become impossible. He recognized that his lack of attention was not only due to short articles with an endless array of hyperlinks. The actual medium of the screen betrayed his focus. So the tech writer did two unthinkable things: he unplugged, then wrote a book about it.

Why write a book when the medium itself seems so outdated? Over the last two decades, books have become more business cards than conscious acts of literature. Plenty of writers remain devoted to the craft of the word, but unless you're in the elitist of the elite, earning a living from this discipline is onerous. Modern writing programs teach you to not use complex sentences requiring critical thinking while assaulting the reader with bold headlines, bullet points, pictures, and floating boxes to keep their brains occupied. Instead of staring at row upon row of text, much better it is to offer eye candy, quotes, and self-affirmations than anything of substance. This is what the reader wants, so make your point and get out, as quickly as possible.

In *The Shallows: What the Internet is Doing to Our Brains*, Carr explores the ways in which this particular medium—the Internet—is altering our ability to think, and subsequently feel, more than any other technological advance in history. We don't often consider the printing press technological, but when Johannes Gutenberg advanced upon a technique that had been evolving in China for nearly 400 years, his moveable press was widely frowned upon. Shifting from handwritten texts to reams of paper rushing through a metal grinder was going to be the downfall of humanity, claimed his critics.

Even the act of writing was deemed an epic failure of the imagination. Crude forms of accounting had been kept on stones and sheets of papyrus for centuries. High art demanded the rigors of memorization. In India oral recitation was king: all 100,000 *shloka* (verse couplet), some 1.8 million Sanskrit words, comprise the entirety of the *Mahābhārata* —more than ten times the length of the *Iliad* and the *Odyssey* combined. As with Homer's epics, poets had to memorize this prose. This trend lives on with imams and mullahs who recite the Qur'an and Shakespearean actors devoted to the bard's works, though neither are mainstream endeavors by any means.

In today's world of tweeting and Instagramming, who would ever be able to retrieve a string of nearly two million words? Granted, such prose rhymed to exploit our brain's penchant for chunking, filing information in groups to make recalling it easier. This might work with a few hundred lines in the twenty-first century, perhaps a TED-sized talk. Given how many yoga classes I've taken in which the instructor forgets a series of eight poses from one side to the other, I'm not confident in total recall.

Then again, our brains are not wired for recalling much of *anything*. We don't even have one type of memory. There's implicit memory, the type in which 'practice makes perfect,' or perhaps better stated, repetition makes a consciously directed action unconscious: tying your shoelaces, riding a bicycle, driving to the café for your morning java. When a person suffers from dementia or Alzheimer's disease, they may very well be able to function such tasks with no problem at all, offering the illusion of self-sufficiency.

Explicit memory is what elders lose when the onset of these diseases occur. One of the two divisions, semantic memory, allows us to learn new things, remember people after we've met them, and gives meaning to the jumble of words we know as sentences. There is no clear dividing line on what makes something implicit or explicit other than what we choose to focus on. The patterns we practice every day most likely fall into the implicit category, while remembering what kind of cake we had at our thirtieth birthday celebration will be more challenging. We'll remember the vague contours of a party while details likely escape us.

Many of us think we have incredible memories. I used to until I realized I don't. At the very least it's selective: I can remember the name of obscure African musicians from the 1970's thanks to my passion for international music, yet I can meet someone five times and not remember their name. This last example helps explain the demise of one aspect of consolidation, an understanding of how memory works that has dominated psychology for decades.

Our brains are comprised of an extremely complex network of neurons—some 100 billion—communicating with one another by propagating an electrical current that travels along a tube-like channel called an axon. The current runs into another neuron at the tip, the synapse, causing the release of a chemical molecule, or the transmitter. For example, a neuron colliding with a muscle fiber results in movement. Interestingly, neurons are not necessary for the sustaining of life—plants are unable to form neurons—but they play a critical role in the creation of the brain phenomenon we call consciousness, of which the storage and retrieval of memories plays a critical component in the formation of our identity.

The old paradigm of consolidation treated memory like a notebook. You jot down an idea or a poem; once the ink is dry, the memory is eternal, save the onset of disease. There is a brief window where you might smudge the ink, making everything hazy. Once the ink is dry, your brain locked that memory in. I've heard people refer to recalling past events like opening a file cabinet and pulling out the folder, which fits neatly along these lines. Only it isn't true.

A 2003 study of 569 college students discovered that 73% of them remembered watching footage of the first plane hitting the World Trade Center on September 11, 2001. The only problem is that no such footage was shown until the following morning. The students were rewriting their narrative to tell a version of the story they wanted to recite, not what actually happened. They were not consciously deceiving researchers. Their recalling of that day had changed, making memory a much more fluid process than we had imagined. Our notebook is more like an Etch a Sketch.

Another outdated manner of looking at memory is described by Antonio Damasio as our eyes and brain working together as a video camera: our eyes passively record events while our brain, also passively, commits the experience to tape. This fits the filing cabinet, or rather hard drive, theory of mind. You dump the footage in, where it remains until you pull the file out.

Memory is in fact an *interaction* with the events and people recorded. Damasio notes that beyond the visual structure of the encounter, the following are also pertinent in the consolidation process: the movements of eyes, neck, and the entire body of those involved; any sensorimotor pattern of touching or engaging with an object or person; any memories evoked during the creation of the memory linking it to previous experiences; emotions induced while experiencing the event.

Memories, then, are composite pictures of you in relation to an object or event, immediately prejudiced by your history and belief system. During every new event you carry with you the entirety of prior experiences. Hence, we all have very different reckonings of places in time. For example, a Muslim listening to an imam declare that women are a secondary species, or an evangelical preacher discussing the sins of same-sex marriage, will feel justified thinking the way they do, while in both situations I would feel a visceral sense of disgust.

Every time you extract a memory, it is put together piecemeal, not as a whole. It is also colored by every experience you have had since that time. The idea of 'perfect memory' is impossible, except for those rare people who have what is known as 'superior memories.' One woman, Jill Price, recalls with startling accuracy every day since 1977. For most of us, what is recalled is subject to the narrative we're trying to explain at that moment, open to the whims of personal decisions we've made as well as the context in which we're retelling it.

Here's the really fascinating part: when we commit something to memory, it is first stored in our short-term memory before being consolidated in long-term memory, mostly while we're asleep. When we retrieve a long-term memory, it does not, as mentioned, come back whole. It also does not remain in long-term parking. It becomes a short-term memory again, and has to go through the process of consolidation all over again, including the generation of proteins necessary in creating new synaptic terminals. This is how we strengthen memories, by constantly recalling them and putting them through the rigorous process of re-remembering over and over.

This is very useful for, say, memorizing nearly two million words of Sanskrit text. On the flip side, this tragic loop keeps us mired in depression and anxiety when dealing with a break-up or the death of a loved one. Corresponding body states associated with the memory are also recalled. We subject ourselves to the negative consequences of increased cortisol and shallow breathing when reminding ourselves of the love we no longer have, which leads to all sorts of spirals, included an increased risk of inflammation and compromising of our immune system, as well as opening ourselves to substance addictions, all due to the *way* we remember.

Holding on to too much is not how we want to live. Yet there are all sorts of dangers with using our technologies as an outsourced memory terminal. The very act of typing instead of handwriting text appears to adversely affect our ability to remember information. It also seems that reading on devices like a Kindle, Nook, or computer screen impairs our ability to consolidate information as compared to that old-fashioned page-turner acquired from your favorite brick-and-mortar.

Nicolas Carr relates memory as the process of filling a bathtub with thimbles of water. The slow, steady pace book readers are accustomed to allow information to be consolidated at a stable rate, making recall easier and more reliable. When we're constantly devouring little bits of text from here and there, our brain is frantically attempting to transfer the meaning of the words, though only committing a small portion to long-term memory. The single-minded concentration, what in yoga we call *ekagrata*, offered by books is lost in the deluge of tweets and updates. Unfortunately that is not all that is lost in the process.

IT MIGHT SEEM CHALLENGING to consider emotions as survival mechanisms. As advanced as we've become in so many realms, we cling to the archaic notion that our 'mind' is something good at arithmetic and following cooking instructions, while the mystical realm known as 'emotions' transcends the functions of the brain. One popular phrase I've heard repeatedly in yoga classes is: 'I am not this body, I am not this mind.' The truth is that you are, and it's nothing to be ashamed of.

Take disgust, which we'll explore in depth in Chapter Nine. This emotion arose as a way of warning us to not eat putrid food. The smell and taste of rotting meat or vegetables kept us from getting sick and dying. Disgust also set social norms—emotions are both individual and social, helping create boundaries as a culture. When someone partakes in an act we find disgusting, such as a farmer having sex with an animal he's milking, the groundwork for ethics is laid.

The longstanding Cartesian split between mind and body is quickly losing traction thanks to advancements in neuroscience. Emotions and thoughts are not necessarily separate from one another. When we speak about emotions, we are usually considering the *feeling* provoked. Primordial feelings are generally unconscious acts in which our body warns us if homeostasis is being achieved. If something goes wrong with our digestion or blood pressure, our body *feels* a certain way, letting our consciousness know that we should visit a doctor. Different feelings invoke different mental responses.

Let's look at one of the most important emotions we possess. The development of empathy has been critical in the survival of our species. Being clued in to how others feel allows us to offer comfort and support, an act sometimes abandoned in the online world. The neural mechanisms underneath empathy and caring—the brainstem, hypothalamus and amygdala—allow us to process first-hand emotional experiences by understanding what another is feeling. Nowhere is this more visible than in a mother caring for her child.

We are all equipped with an urge to nurture. We might say the roots of compassion reach deep into the ancient circuits of maternal devotion. A symphony of emotions exists between mother and infant. The same neural networks and brain pathways activated during empathy drive the nurturing and compassionate instinct, yet it is the production of oxytocin that generates the strong love between mother and baby. We might later assign a mystical aspect to this love, and there's not much harm if it helps us care for our child better. But don't confuse the point: oxytocin is the chemical responsible.

Neuroscientist Richard J. Davidson decided to see if a higher emotion such as compassion has a neural correlate. His brain scans revealed significant activity in the insula, a region near the brain's frontal portion that plays a key role in bodily representations of emotion, and the same area activated in empathy research. Activity also increased in the temporal parietal juncture, particularly the right hemisphere. Studies have implicated this area as important in processing empathy, especially in perceiving the mental and emotional state of others. The circumstances in which we display empathy and compassion might vary; the brain region activated is the same.

I've often heard empathy and compassion regarded as yogic goals. The art of compassion, something Buddha heralded as a high state of achievement, implies that not only do you recognize the suffering of another person, but that you also lend a hand to help him overcome it. This sense of selflessness succinctly captures an elemental foundation of modern yoga, and it could be the prime example of mental or emotional purity: the brilliant dance of conscious action and brain chemistry. If there is any practice of *saucha* I'd like to see implemented more widely, it is this.

We're losing a critical piece of this equation in our allegiance to the technologies purportedly bringing us together. Whenever I spy a yoga teacher taking a photo of the class she is teaching for Instagram, or when I share a meal with someone who spends more time on their device than making eye contact, I wonder how the chemical bonds of empathy can be strengthened. In truth, they cannot be. Not only does distraction help destroy the purity of relationships, it tears at the fabric of our intelligence and emotional response systems.

Let's consider one more example of this neural deficiency. I have a number of friends who rely on talking GPS devices to get everywhere. Granted, Los Angeles is a complicated city to travel in. Last year I regularly had business meetings with a friend in the Miracle Mile district. Every time I rode with him he turned on his machine to navigate. I asked him once to go from memory; he immediately replied that he couldn't. Ironically, there were only two main roads necessary for getting there. Because he waited for the voice instead of paying attention to his surroundings, he was never quite sure where he was.

This seemingly innocuous trend has far-reaching consequences. A landmark study in the late 1990's found that London cab drivers that had memorized the city's map boasted an enlarged posterior hippocampus, important for storing and manipulating spatial surroundings. The longer the driver had been working, the larger that brain region. Unsurprisingly, as drivers rely more on GPS, their ability to memorize anything deteriorates.

Having to memorize one thing does not distract from recalling something else. In fact, it strengthens it. As Carr writes, when we rely on the Internet and our devices instead of personal memory, we are not allowing our brains to consolidate, which will in the end make it challenging to remember anything. This 'ecosystem of interruption technologies,' as journalist Cory Doctorow dubbed them, is helping to destroy our humanity.

That's because it's not only memory being affected. Our aptitude for engaging in empathy and compassion is also suffering.

Today we might read faster than ever, as Carr mentions, but we no longer retain the information long enough to piece together seemingly disparate elements of a bigger story. As he writes, "The strip-mining of 'relevant content' replaces the slow excavation of meaning."

The more we strive for the quick release of dopamine from the smartphone ding, the increased number of times we nervously check our phone when standing in line 'doing nothing'—French café culture should be in uproar over the demise of people watching—or, worse, texting while driving, the more we train our brains in the sad art of distraction. The ability to engage in 'deep thinking,' the slowly excavated process that requires a sharp sense of focus, is eroding our intelligence, and, most tragically, our ability to care about others.

"It's not only deep thinking that requires a calm, attentive mind," Carr writes. "It's also empathy and compassion. Psychologists have long studied how people experience fear and react to physical threats, but it's only recently that they've begun researching the sources of our nobler instincts. What they're finding is that…the higher emotions emerge from neural processes that 'are inherently slow.'"

The wedding of thought and emotion. Our toys are playing us.

Numerous yoga instructors have said that yoga returns us to our 'original state,' one they often believe entails happiness, contentment, compassion and inner peace. I disagree. At birth we are dependent more than anything else. We depend on the care and attention of others to survive, and not only for our first five or so years on earth. It would be nice to imagine that we were 'originally' peaceful and serene. In reality our brains are anything but. Those are habits we have to train for and implement, not a default condition of the human species.

If we want to attain cleanliness of thought and being, we cannot be constantly distracted. We won't end up there magically, through a few yoga classes when *savasana* leaves us 'blissed out.' We have to fight the ravages of our brains—the *I'm not good enough*, the *I'll do it later*, the *That doesn't really matter*—every step of the way. This requires an abandoning of habits, like the one I opened this chapter with. When our social intelligence drops a few points because everyone is looking at their screen instead of the road in front of us, we've lost something important. When in the same process we lose the ability to truly care for others, we have to start to wonder just what being human means in the first place, and whether this primordial connection is worth the sacrifice.

4 APARIGRAHA : LETTING GO

IMAGINE YOU ARE LYING in bed, awake. It's two am. The sounds around you: a door closing, floorboards creaking, wind against the window. Your ears scan for something more remote. Then, a skid. Could it be? You're not certain. The adrenalin rush ensures you'll be awake at least another hour, probably two.

Sirens follow. A fire truck is first on the scene—you've well learned the differences between blares. You jump out of bed, slip on a brand new pair of sneakers and are out the door before the first police siren whirls. Within four minutes you're parked a block away, red and blue and white lights forcing your pupils to dilate quicker than you'd like at this late hour. Early hour.

You watch policemen question the stunned driver, his car wrapped around a telephone pole. He is disoriented though not fatally shaken. Perhaps drunk. The ambulance arrives, stretches out a cot. He disappears as the truck's jaws close. The firemen depart soon after. A tow truck pulls the totaled sedan onto a flatbed, drives away, followed by the police. Debris is scattered, a job for the cleaning crew, which doesn't arrive at work until eight. You have plenty of time.

Broken headlights, shards of chipped grill, flecks of black paint—none of these interest you. You grab a flashlight to scan the cement for puddles of fluid: oil, gasoline, windshield wiper, brake, battery. Especially the latter. An oblong slick curves toward the curb. You rush to your trunk, emerging with a gallon of heavy-duty soap and a metallic brush. You clean. Obsessively.

Obsessively, for this is what you do every night. Your insomnia is dictated by the siren calls of fire engines and medical workers, on the lucky nights. Most evenings you lie awake in anticipation, your desire to cleanse roads of acid and oil denied by a lack of mortal wounds.

You drive home after being satisfied the scrubbing is sufficient. On the way inside you toss your sneakers into the garbage can. Once sunlight arrives you'll purchase another pair, for who knows what awaits you when the sun dips below the horizon once again. You fall asleep, briefly, and start the cycle again.

APARIGRAHA MEANS 'GREEDLESSNESS,' or non-grasping. It originates from the word *parigraha*, claiming something for yourself. Like all Sanskrit words, adding an 'a' in front creates its antonym. Patanjali writes that when practiced to perfection, *aparigraha* leads to knowledge of your own birth. More widespread is its usage in giving up possessions: it is the *yama* fueling the ascetic movement, men tired of householder life ready to become one with god or nature or whatever lurks in the forest.

Just how ascetic one must be is a matter of opinion. In the *Bhagavad Gītā* Krishna implores yogis to abandon all belongings, which is why you'll find roadside sadhus begging for alms, owning nothing more than the dhoti wrapped around their midsection. Other texts, such as the *Bhāgavata Purāna*, state that you should only own what is necessary and nothing more. While nowhere near a call for extreme asceticism, such an interpretation would certainly challenge the modern American.

When investigated in terms of property, *asteya* and *aparigraha* are cousins if not siblings. Stealing and greed go hand-in-hand. In this chapter I'm going to look at another definition: non-grasping. The grasping of thoughts is a greed all its own, one we're not always capable of controlling, as in the example of the man who spent every night awaiting car accidents described above. While a more drastic example of habitual patterning known as obsessive-compulsive disorder, it is nonetheless a true story.

OCD is a powerful example of how our brain operates. The disorder can range from excessive hand washing (a trademark of the disease) to manically peering into your rearview mirror every time your car hits a bump in fear that you've just run over someone. Symptoms vary from mild annoyance (Oh, that's just Ken brushing his teeth ten times a day) to outright dangerous (Ken's brushing habit has permanently damaged his gums and ruined his marriage). The most popular compulsions are to wash and check; the fear of microbes and bacteria overwhelms, as does the urge to ensure nothing is amiss, such as the proverbial stove left on. Our brains can cripple us if we don't have the proper guidance for dealing with its treacherous mechanisms.

Even if you do not have OCD, everyone has experienced the fixation of certain thoughts. As we explored in the last chapter, memories moved from short-term storage to long-term holding are ones we invoke over and over. By continually transferring a memory from long- to short-term, we strengthen the neural connections making that memory 'real.' While there are assorted levels of obsessiveness, all habits are based on neurons continually firing together. The more we think it, the more we believe it.

This is how we become 'stuck,' trapped in a pattern. Consider your morning coffee. The freezer opening, aroma of beans, procedural scooping into a machine—or, if you're like me, an AeroPress—the bubbling and gurgling of water, steam rising as the grounds are transformed, transforming you from groggy to alert. This is one of the most popular rituals in the world, and for good reason: it appeals to a number of our senses. It is also an addiction, albeit one with debatable consequences. (I lean toward the health aspects, but I'm biased.)

Now don't have your morning coffee. You are certain to be

irritable, imagining the taste of the bitter liquid in your mouth, the slow sips, quick awakening, flutter of heart palpitations. Most likely a headache ensues, if not that morning then definitely the next. Beyond the caffeine detox is the habitual hold of the wired neurons impatiently tapping an imaginary finger in wait of their fix.

We like to compartmentalize our experiences. When things run smoothly, we barely even notice the regular functions of the day. We teach ourselves that A always precedes B. Then one day B jumps up and takes the lead. Your entire world is amiss. Someone cut your espresso supply without warning.

I personally witnessed this on September 11, 2001. I left for work early, getting on the PATH train at Exchange Place in Jersey City shortly before eight am. My commute had me exiting at the World Trade Center four minutes later, taking the A train to my gym before work. While all memories fade and rearrange, I distinctly recall leaving the gym to walk north, noticing dozens of people standing in the middle of Sixth Ave gazing south. I turned. B jumped in front of A; a nation's understanding of reality flipped.

It was hard for people to understand that what happened that morning has been going down in other countries for centuries. This does not make it right; it only intensifies our sting. After briefly checking in at my office, I walked from 36th St and Ninth Ave to 91st St and First Ave to my then-girlfriend's apartment. Along the way I passed through Times Square.

Recall the opening scene of *I Am Legend*. Will Smith walks through a desolate, deserted Times Square, save a runaway lion. I'm pretty certain the director was there on 9/11. There were no cars; people walked aimlessly along the avenues, in the same daze I was in. Then the oddest thing occurred. I walked by a shoe store. It was *packed*. As in it could barely hold another customer. While most businesses were shut down, this single store was hitting a sales record. People were holding three, four, six boxes while understaffed workers scurried about.

We may never know why in the midst of the greatest terrorist attack in recent American history people felt it necessary to purchase shoes. Some might have needed more appropriate footwear to walk over New York City bridges since public transportation was shut down. Yet that wouldn't explain six boxes. There is more to it. Shopping provides comfort to some. What's your first inclination after a break-up, a raise or even having a productive day? Reward yourself, which often includes purchasing an object. What was one of the first things President Bush encouraged good Americans to do in the days after 9/11? Shop! Keep our economy strong by buying things!

This is how engrained habits are. Even during a national tragedy we reverted to our basest impulses. Sadly, in this case, it involved credit cards.

There are ways to work through such impulses and change habitual patterns, or what in yoga are known as *samskāras*, 'activators' or mental imprints that set us into action. If something can be grasped, if it can be possessed, it is certainly within our power to ungrasp it, to let it go. First, let's explore one intriguing piece of this puzzle helping to facilitate the wiring and rewiring of our brains.

'ATTENTION. ATTENTION.' So called the mynah birds, day after day, at first surprising then soothing the shipwrecked Will Farnaby in Aldous Huxley's *Island*, the author's 1962 counterpart to *Brave New World*. Landing on the remote island of Pala, Farnaby watches as this Mahayana Buddhist society reckons with outside forces industrializing the nation. Farnaby treats this promised futuristic utopia cynically and empathically, constantly brought back into the moment by the shrill cry of the island's birds, themselves perhaps the only true proponents of Buddhism in the book.

Is constant attention even possible? It would be wonderful to always be 'in the moment,' yet what of that wonderful tool called the imagination? Are daydreams counterproductive, or can we let our minds roam freely?

It comes down to one simple word: play.

As discussed in Chapter One, Jaak Panksepp treats play as a primary process embedded deep in the oldest parts of our brain. It is an evolutionary and social tool: play teaches us boundaries within our group. This is why more joy emanates from adults who are playful in their outlook of life, compared to those carrying the serious weight of existence on their shoulders. It also explains our fascination with sci-fi adventure movies and shows: *Lord of the Rings, Star Wars, Game of Thrones.* We are emotionally invested in these ongoing sagas thanks to the incredible characters as well as the human truths revealed, even when presented in distant and future cultures far (yet somehow not so far) away.

Play did not just arise with Tolkien or Spielberg. In India, *leela* (or *lilā*) describes the manner in which existence came to be. Translating as 'play,' *leela* is the perpetual dance of the cosmos holding the universe together, symbolized by Shiva in Dancer's pose, or Natraj. This many-armed deity represents play in its destructive form. The dance destroys illusions so new worlds can be reconstructed. In a more romantic light, *leela* is Krishna playing his flute for *gopis*, shepherdesses, multiplying himself to make every young lass believe that he was serenading her alone.

The world is a spontaneous creation requiring a fusion of positive and negative attributes to be sustained. This is *leela* according to non-dual schools. It also represents, as Alan Watts noticed, an important cultural rift: in the West, God is detached, predominantly absent, except when he arrives to display His endless anger. Across the ocean gods dance and laugh among humans, play informing them as to how the universe operates. They don't finger wag. They finger wrestle.

For *leela* to give form to the formless, another element is necessary. The word *maya* is often translated as 'illusion,' but as Professor of Religions William K. Mahony points out, a more fitting definition is 'magic creative force.' In this sense *maya* is the evolutionary force behind everything we experience, the process pushing us along. The same tool inspiring us to write mythologies and epic stories helps create everything we see: buildings, roads, wireless networks, this book you hold in your hands, whatever we have ever dreamed into being. Though maya is a function of the gods, according to Indian philosophy it is available to humans when using our imagination.

In the yoga traditions I've studied, imagination and meditation are at odds. While there is nothing inherently bad about the former, yogis are told to focus on one thing for an extended period of time, such as breathing, a mantra or a candle's flame. The idea is to become dissolved in the present moment so thoroughly that a 'blowing out,' or nirvana, of your individual identity occurs. Engulfed by the present you realize there is no distance between the universe and yourself; it all intertwines and works together as one continuous process. There is nothing wrong with this form of meditation. It just turns out other ways work as well.

A recent study conducted in Norway revealed intriguing results with nondirective meditation. Instead of intensely attempting to focus on a single object, meditators simply closed their eyes and let their brains go in whatever direction it wanted, not consciously attempting to control anything. This practice showed increased activity in their hippocampus and amygdala, the centers for episodic memory and emotional processing. It appears letting your brain 'go' aids your ability to remember as well as deal with emotional situations. This does not discount directive meditation, which has been proven to have many positive neural and emotional benefits. It does, however, make you wonder why your grade school teacher told you to stop daydreaming, as if the lands you visited in your mind offered no benefits whatsoever. (Granted, context is crucial. Taking your attention off the road to look at your phone is not an example of nondirective attention.)

Another aspect of play is happening all the time, in your home, at work, in your car: musicians playing together. Music clues us in on how our brains operate when in a playful state. The word *raga* (from classical Indian music) means 'color.' Music was thought to color the world, giving rise to empathy, passion, and all the other drives it produces within us. A musician 'plays' their instrument to produce these colors that light up our imagination, triggering a wide array of emotions and invoking memories as we constantly update our life's soundtrack.

People moving together with the sole purpose of having fun and feeling good, as you might see in a dance club or by watching musicians on stage, elicit a connection with music and play dating back to ancient times. Both seem optional to human existence, yet there appears to be a biological utility as well. Dancing and performing music promote positive emotions through brain chemistry, social interaction, and in the physiology of arousing our body to move. They are pleasurable experiences as well, energizing and enlivening us while offering the opportunity to let go from the burden of everyday life. Music and play renew any lost sense of optimism and open us up to a new world of possibilities.

Both music and play affect the processes of the brain that reward us with pleasure. They allow us to engage fully with others and feel a deep emotional connection. Language is unnecessary in enjoying the full benefits of either. Because of this scientists believe that music is not only a precursor to language, but evolved out of natural playful activities. Your friend grunts; you follow, mimicking the noise (as mimicry is one way we learn and connect). Soon you're slapping your thighs in a rudimentary rhythm, your friend joins in, howling overtop. A bond through sound, the rush of dopamine and oxytocin causing you to want to do it again and again.

In the same way that opioids and pleasure hormones like serotonin are released when listening to music, playing unleashes the same chemicals and hormones. Neuroscientists, developmental psychologists, biologists, and many other researchers from every area of the scientific world understand play as a profound biological process. It has evolved over eons in many animals to promote survival. It shapes the brain and helps make animals smarter and more adaptable. It also fosters bonds and empathy and helps bind complex social groups together. For humans, play is at the center of how we learn to build our imagination, creativity, innovation and happiness.

The ancestral sources of social joy and laughter are what Panksepp calls play. He believes PLAY is an emotional system serving as the foundation of joy, a creative means for expressing our imagination. Panksepp also claims that through play we learn how to operate as social animals. The desire to engage and create is fostered through such an attitude. It's no wonder some of our earliest memories occur on the playground, a widespread cultural image reminding us of the freedom of childhood.

Early Indian writers who envisioned a flute-playing Krishna as the binding force of existence were onto something. Evolutionary psychologists, musicologists, anthropologists, and neuroscientists believe music allowed humans to become the complex social animals we are today. Music seems to have strengthened community bonds and helped resolve conflicts. Because music comprehension is possible only in intelligent brains, neuroscientists such as Dan Levitin think music aided in building our brains. Social interaction through music has been the driving force behind the explosion in human brain size.

Professor of Archaeology and Psychology Steve Mithen feels that music was used to build group identity through playing together. Performing and sharing music with others facilitate bonds between familial, social and even disparate parties. Performance affords us the opportunity to connect. While in no way a replacement for the sharing of live music with others, online groups and message boards offer a different sense of connection as bands use social media to build community. Feeling invested in those who create the music you love adds another layer of enjoyment and fulfillment in the entire play process.

Play is, of course, not a solitary endeavor. Research has shown that we are thirty times more likely to laugh with another person or in a group. While our imagination is indeed of our own doing, it must be played out in the theater of community. Having a vision is the first step on a journey that by necessity includes others.

Since we are group-oriented, the possibility of grasping lessens: you don't only think about yourself when resources are shared. Odd as it sounds, this is sometimes one of the harder lessons to understand. It's easy to be sucked back into habitual patterns that place personal survival (or desires) ahead of the group, a trend more common in America than a number of other cultures. Research between Americans and East Asians showed this to be the case. When asked to write twenty statements using the term "I," Americans overwhelmingly wrote things like 'happy,' 'outgoing,' and 'interested in jazz,' all descriptions of their personal preferences and attitudes. By contrast, East Asians listed their relationships and roles in society: 'son,' 'wife,' 'employee.'

Developing a playful attitude while recognizing that your actions and desires affect others, and not only those in your group, is one way to counteract and, hopefully, transform greediness into something more sustainable and considerate of others.

Every light casts its shadow, however. The human imagination is one of the most powerful aspects of this evolutionary trait we call consciousness, and for millennia we have used it for amazing purposes. Yet it has also paralyzed individuals in one very unfortunate way: the conspiracy theory.

NO PLANES EVER HIT the World Trade Center. It was an intricate plot designed by the ~~US government Bush cartel GOP conspiring with the Taliban~~ Illuminati to get ~~foreign oil American consumers to buy more~~ aliens into high positions of government. These are the same architects who conspired to fool us into thinking ~~Sandy Hook Benghazi gay marriage the Boston Marathon~~ the Aurora murders were real and not just crisis actors portraying roles they were paid for. That and, oh, ~~Sudan Mali the Congo global warming~~ the Holocaust never happened. Area 51 for life.

The Internet has assisted the proliferation of conspiracy

theories. Here's the thing: conspiracies *are* real. They do happen. In the past they were much easier to get away with. Governments really harm its own citizens. Mexican journalist Anabel Hernández has been living under armed protection since publishing her groundbreaking 2010 book, *Los Señores del Narco* (*Narcoland: The Mexican Drug Lords and their Godfathers*), which exposed the national government's collusion with drug cartels. In our own country Edward Snowden revealed years of governmental spying on innocent civilians. We cannot trust everything we're told.

Skepticism is a healthy trait, one investigate journalists like Hernández need to make use of. There's a difference between a woman who has dedicated decades of her life to intense research and someone sitting at their computer for too long stumbling across a doctored picture with a pyramid in it. Such ease of communication has led to too much bad information. Since all it takes is a click to share a story, there's no need to even read the content or investigate whether or not that content is real. Conspiracy theorists are intense contrarians. In their world, everything is a hoax and nothing is ever to be taken for what it is.

Thinking 'the game' is rigged against you, always, is not healthy. What's worse, it damages us culturally. An April, 2013, poll revealed that 37% of Americans think global warming is nonsense despite decades of scientific research to the contrary. Twenty-eight percent believe an Illuminati-type secret society bides its time until world domination is complete, while 21% of US citizens are certain that our government is hiding aliens.

In the technical sense, conspiracy theories are not actually theories. The rigorous investigatory process in scientific studies is absent. Logic often has to be suspended in order to cobble together the looniest ideas. Conflicting data is not a hindrance; sometimes it's a badge of honor, showing the extreme lengths that 'evil powers that be' go in covering up wrongdoing. Specificities are mostly irrelevant if the tale fits into a larger narrative. If a person is liable to believe in one conspiracy theory, Pandora's box has been opened. They'll fall for others.

A 2008 study found that people who buy into conspiracy theories had difficulties with emotional processing, a trait associated with the amygdala. Innate feelings of powerlessness and uncertainty are markers of those scanning the Internet for controversies. It exploits our brain's necessity for filling in gaps, an evolutionary survival technique. That cognitive lesson has translated, in the digital age, into writing a narrative for every tale, no matter how far-fetched or impossible. If you are generally fearful of life, your imagination will be guided by such fears, making conspiracy theories attractive. We are not only what we think. We create reality by whatever patterns of thought we've bought into.

This becomes dangerous when political activists, for one, use this cognitive dissonance to their advantage. Suddenly everything becomes a controversy concocted by the Obama administration to do harm to American citizens. Levelheaded Republicans are ousted in primaries, which generally see low turnout and appeal to fringe voters. Congressional policies making us shake our head in disbelief are the result of this insidious agenda. This, for one, is not a conspiracy. You only need to witness the results of local elections for verification. Whenever you ask yourself 'how did that guy get into office?' check out his platform and observe who those ideas appealed to. Powerlessness and power often go hand in hand.

Conspiracies begin with a thought, one suiting those who feel disempowered. Powers are against you, but you know the truth. You justify your thoughts by finding groups of like-minded citizens online or at rallies. An intense feedback loop of disinformation develops. Your small community is bolstered by the belief that all small communities hold the keys to truth. Oppression and laughter directed at you become badges of honor indicating that you've uncovered epic truths. Feelings of rightness become addictive, a form of grasping, bringing us back to where we started.

MANY PEOPLE CANNOT WILL something away. Consciously invoking a deep-seated fear or addiction is not a healthy path to recovery. The idea of 'cold turkey' works for some; as a form of general therapy results are dismal. UCLA psychiatrist Jeffrey Schwartz notes that the behaviorist approach to treating OCD in the eighties damaged more patients than it cured. Psychiatrists would take patients obsessed with cleaning to public bathrooms and make them wipe their hands on toilets, even smearing parts of their bodies after touching the bowls. Then they would be prevented from going to the sink.

Besides being an obvious sanitary disaster, Schwartz writes that roughly 30% of patients wouldn't even go so far as to step into the bathroom. If you can't even begin to implement a cure, chances of recovery are nil. While Schwartz's ideas on mind-body dualism are suspect, his four-step program to recovery, a blend of cognitive therapy, Buddhist mindfulness and Viennese economic theory, has successfully helped many patients:

- Relabel: Identify deceptive brain messages and the uncomfortable feelings they invoke and immediately treat them for what they are.
- Reframe: Treat them as 'false brain messages' in order to change your perception of what they truly are.
- Refocus: Direct your perception toward a productive mental process or activity. If you have a thought about washing your hands, pick up the sweater you're knitting or go out to the garden instead.
- Revalue: Give the deceptive thoughts no value (the part pulled from economics) while recognizing them as sensations and not reflections of reality.

Schwartz recognized that behavioral therapies were treating humans like automata. When brain scans showed OCD specific to three brain regions—the orbital frontal cortex, caudate nucleus and anterior cingulate gyrus—he knew that if he changed the chemical behavior in these regions, he could help patients rewire their neural circuitry. He likens this chemical dance to driving: the caudate nucleus was failing to perform its gating function, what he compares to a 'sticky manual transmission.' Because of this a direct pathway between thoughts is impossible, as the patient cannot move on to the next thought. He termed this phenomenon 'brain lock.' A person hones in on one obsessive thought in a deadly feedback loop, unable to move on. Schwartz's four-step solution is designed to disrupt this chain.

Schwartz's disruption is still applicable for those of us who do not suffer from OCD. First we have to understand how habits form. Habits are usually viewed as specific actions, but they are actually part of a continuum of human behavior, according to professors Ann M. Graybiel and Kyle S. Smith. We only have a certain amount of cognitive space for attention, which is why recent studies have shown how mentally unhealthy multitasking is. Behaviors become automatic so we don't have to keep putting the same amount of attention into the actions: riding a bike, driving a car, brushing your teeth and so on. The more routine a behavior becomes, the less attention we pay to it. That's how bad habits become so normal that we don't even recognize them as unhealthy. They're simply part of our everyday.

The extreme end of this is OCD, though certain habits are more insidious: substance abuse, computer gaming, constantly checking your phone. Traits exploiting our brain's pleasure-reward system overtake us; they don't seem abnormal at all. The habit has become engrained. I sometimes challenge my students by asking them to not check their phone the next time they have the impulse and see if they feel an anxious rush or notice their hand shaking. Then they'll know if their habit has moved into the realm of addiction.

That is not a therapy, however. Just as Schwartz noticed, telling yourself not to do something does not equate to a change in behavior. Our brains are accustomed to the dollop of pleasure associated with an action. If we resist and nothing is there to replace it, the alternative (not checking your phone) is not going to be reinforced as something positive. Behind the scenes of consciousness our brains are valuing every action in terms of the reward it brings.

Studies conducted in Australia on rats, humans, and monkeys found habitual behavior linked to activity in the striatum and basal ganglia interconnecting the neocortex. At the beginning of one experiment, neurons in the striatum dealing with motor control were highly active. Once a skill was learned (in this case rats running a course through a maze) those neurons remained highly active only at the beginning and end of the quest. They were quiet during most of the regimen, much how we don't pay attention when we're tying our shoes. Graybiel and Smith relate this to our tendency to chunk information: remembering a phone number in longer strings of numbers rather than one by one. This is also why Indian mythologies rhymed and, as mentioned, the 'a' at the beginning denotes a Sanskrit word's opposite. Our brain seeks the easiest possible route to information. Researchers believe the striatum chunks information by helping us "combine a sequence of action into one unit."

Habit-related circuits in the striatum gain strength the more an activity is repeated. Interestingly, in the learning process there is very little activity in the infralimbic cortex, located near the front of the neocortex. Only after a habit is formed by the striatum is information then chunked in the neocortex, as if the former is vetting the reward before allowing the habit to become deeply engrained. Even when an activity seems unconscious, our brain is always monitoring the reward, so that if we diverge from a set pattern, we're certain to know about it. Hello caffeine headaches.

At this time there is no silver bullet for breaking habitual patterns. Schwartz's four-step program does provide a good blueprint for anyone trying to overcome damaging patterns. Graybiel and Smith offer their own suggestions: removing the candy dish from eyesight or keeping a pair of running shoes next to the bed for when you wake up in the morning. Of course if you're waking up at midnight to scrub the street, a different course of action might be necessary.

The tendrils of grasping are inherent in all of us. We are never going to be without habits. Best to use them for our benefit while doing as little harm as possible to those around us. Otherwise we're holding tightly to something guaranteed to slip away.

While on the Asian Massive tour in 2002 I was sitting in a van next to Algerian-born DJ Cheb i Sabbah, who unfortunately passed from cancer in November, 2013. We were talking about yoga, as his Indian-based electronic albums include some of the best modern music for the practice I've ever heard. He was frustrated by the evolution of the business and marketing of yoga, what he called 'spirituality for sale.' When we moved onto the idea of addiction and using yoga in recovery, he said, "Now of course it's better to do yoga than to smoke crack."

I'll never forget his wisdom or his smile, or the truth behind his offhand mysticism. We need to choose our habits well.

5 BRAHMACHARYA : SELF-HONESTY

BABULAL GAUR YADAV knows how to get elected. He also understands how to stay in power. The Uttar Pradesh native has been voted into ten Assembly elections in his native India, a record for the man who resides over Govindpura in Bhopal. A former Chief Minister in his state, he is currently responsible for maintaining law and order.

Babulal was born into the Ahir community—many consider the Ahirs and Yadavs to be synonymous. (Like the Bauls, some ethnic groups in India have the same last name. You'll see this in the Kundalini yoga community when Americans adopt either Singh or Kaur, from the Sikh tradition. It is a tribal practice linking members of the same community.) Cattle herders by trade, the Yadav movement has been progressive for at least a century with its attempts of improving social standings through expansion of economic opportunities and by active participation in the armed forces and politics. The eighty-four-year-old Babulal is an example of the latter. In 2018 he will be celebrating a half-century in his seat.

'Progressive' is a relative term, however. While the Yadavs have focused intensely on finances over the last century, other areas remain questionable. Sexual violence is on the rise in India. This reached a climax in May, 2014, when a photo of two teenage girls hanging from a tree in Utter Pradesh after being gang raped went viral. Roughly half of India's 1.25 billion people have no access to toilets. The fields where they relieve themselves are often monitored by men awaiting new victims. In fact, two policemen were said to be involved in the raping of these young girls, who are believed to have hung themselves due to the social disgrace that follows being sexually assaulted.

Think of that: first, you are attacked by a group of men who easily overpower you in a dark field. Then you are subjected to ridicule in your community because of it. On top of this, the protectors prove to be anything but. The head of Utter Pradesh's governing party, Mulayam Singh Yadav, recently opposed a law calling for gang-rapists to be executed. During his statement he commented, "Boys will be boys. They make mistakes."

Apparently Babulal is in alignment with his fellow politician. When asked about the recent gang rapes, he responded, "This is a social crime that depends on men and women. Sometimes it's right, sometimes it's wrong." It's hard to imagine any situation is which rape is 'right.' Yet this attitude toward women has long been part of our evolutionary heritage. It is, fortunately, a stance Americans took great strides in fixing in the twentieth century. I'm not implying we've fully corrected the issue. We still have a lot of work left to do, here and around the world.

BRAHMACHARYA IS PERHAPS THE MOST contested of the *yamas*. While the most ascetic of the claims—complete abstention from sex—is reserved for extreme acolytes, exactly when and how to use one's sexual energy is debated. Some claim it implies sex should only be practiced in a healthy, monogamous relationship, while others say it's not relationship status that matters, but that you only engage in sex wisely, a rather ambiguous term open to wide interpretation. I've heard others claim *brahmacharya* has nothing to do with sex; it is a form of spiritual advancement through inner training. Fair enough, though to claim it does not pertain to sexual conduct, both historically and in the literature, is false.

Brahmacharya translates as 'brahmic conduct,' an upper caste practice implying chastity because, in the eyes of *brahmans*, *brahmans* transcend gender distinctions. This is sort of like saying billionaires transcend financial regulations because billionaires say they do, which has played out in both theory and practice in America. Nevertheless, yogis meditated on the union of male and female energies because great power supposedly resides in semen. If you haven't already noticed, yoga texts are predominantly reserved for men, because it was believed only men really practice yoga.

Even today, as witnessed by the sentiments of Babulal Gaur Yadav, patriarchy still grips part of Indian culture, strains of which are felt in the States. In his *Washington Post* column on June 7, 2014, George Will described new efforts to combat sexual assaults on college campuses as a ploy to "make victimhood a coveted status that confers privilege." Because, of course, 'nonconsensual touching,' as he terms it, is not at all related to rape, and the women attacked in such a manner wear their scars proudly. This disconnection between politicians, policemen, and pundits and the actual public is disturbing, pointing to an inability to come to terms with our very human and very real sexuality and, more importantly, that everyone should be afforded the right to offer or not offer themselves to others.

Patanjali claimed that those practicing *brahmacharya* are endowed with great vitality. This sentiment runs through many societies, some of which demanded that their soldiers not have sex the night before battle as it would deplete vital energy. The *Bhagavad Gita* considered it a form of bodily asceticism, or *tapas*. The *Kurma Purāna* outright banned yogis from sexual intercourse, not just the physical actions, but in mind and speech as well. So did the *Darshana Upanishad*, which claimed the yogi practicing *brahmacharya* would move their mind to that of the *brahman*.

The *Agni Purāna* was much more explicit. You had to renounce all eight degrees of sexual activity: fantasizing; glorifying sex or pretty much anyone of the opposite gender; *looking* at a woman; secretly talking with a woman; dalliance; resolving that you were going to break your vow of chastity; actually having sex; and finally, the saddest of all, longing. Just think of all the beautiful Indian and Sufi poetry that would have been lost to the world if longing, what in Portugal is so gorgeously expressed as *saudade*, was prohibited. The imagination is built for the expression of longing. Yes, yoga is at times a reigning in of the senses, but to deny humans one of the most foundational aspects of our brains and bodies is the perfect set-up for neuroses, which is why longstanding scandals involving priests molesting young boys continue to plague the Church. You deny it, it ravages you.

The *Linga Purāna* is a bit more realistic. While forest dwellers were called upon to practice total abstinence, householders were allowed to partake in sexual relations as long as it involved their wives. This is much more in alignment with what America's religious considers marriage: a sacred vow limiting sexual relations to one partner. That does not mean marriage must follow this particular trajectory. If two consenting adults have worked out what works best for them, alternatives might work. Regardless, sex has long been contemplated, to painful degrees, by thinkers who might have spent too much time working on agendas and not enough experiencing the most elemental (and some would argue, fun) aspect of our and all animal species: the biological drive to continue the lineage.

Equating sex, and its sometimes partner, love, to biology inherently irks some, who like to paint such acts with poetic imagery. While I'm all for the works of Neruda and Rumi, it's important to recognize that almost all of our drives have a biological basis. (Music is one important exception.) Granted, sex as a vehicle for spiritual transmission is, in fact, a pleasurable consequence of this procreative urge, one most dominated in the Western mind by the practice of Tantra. While scholars like the late Georg Feuerstein attempted to remove *Kama Sutra* instructional sex therapy videos from the Tantric lineage, it is impossible to disassociate Tantra from those captivating bodily fluids that have kept yogis enthralled for centuries.

Tantra means 'web' or 'woof,' derived from *tan*, 'to expand.'

The image of an expansive web was deemed a fitting image for the practitioner, who through the practice of Tantra attempted to enlarge his understanding of knowledge, *jnana*. Tantric practices were not created in a vacuum. Like all spiritual disciplines, it was both a social response to growing Brahminic power and a theoretical offshoot of the *Puranas*, the very texts heralding abstinence and the retention of semen. Like many Hindu writings, contradiction is not a bad thing; and like many before and after, sex and violence were at times nearly indistinguishable.

What informed the *Tantras* was mythology, predominantly in the figure of Shiva, the yogic lord who always seems to pop up wherever a paradox is found. While Tantra as its own practice emerged in the sixth century CE (and found its full force in the tenth century), early writings of a proto-Tantra dates back five centuries earlier. Around that time a sage named Lakulisha founded a sect dubbed the Pashupatas, which worshipped Shiva, the Lord of Beasts. The Pashupatas lived in cremation grounds and loved fluids of all kinds: blood, alcohol and the host of sexual juices running unconstrained from ritual intercourse. These early writings were the first to influence what would later become expressed in Tantra.

Disregarding caste laws, the Pashupatas rebelled against their society's 1%, the Brahmins. It was unavoidable that Shiva would eventually kill Brahmins, including their major deity, Brahma. One day Brahma decided to chase after Sarasvati. Shortly after attempting to pick her up, he ran into Shiva, and Brahma's fifth head made a sound that annoyed him. So Shiva cut if off. To his chagrin, it stuck to his hand. The unshakable skull become a sign of his savior status: he had sacrificed his own standing in the eyes of the gods by cutting off the evil head of Brahma, not all that much different than the mythical figure of Jesus, who likewise, through a process of imagined transference, died for the sins of others. By anticipating future sins, Shiva intervened and destroyed an evil sounding head that had just recently attempted to pick up the goddess of music. Hindu deity drama usurps any reality television that we are capable of imagining.

In dedication, the Pashupatas eventually transformed into the Kapalikas, or Skull Bearers. Myth meets life as some devotees, especially those from the lower caste, picked out human skulls to eat their food from. *Bhakti*, devotion, runs strong in such veins. Their deity honors them when he marries even though he had undertaken the chaste vows of the forest wanderer. God meets human. If you're a married householder, you desire a deity cool with sex. Shiva's multiform reality keeps the universe's colorful theatrics in order.

We approach something closer to Tantra in the myth of Sati, one of Shiva's many wives. Her father, Daksha, wasn't feeling this cumbersome yogi who hung out at cemeteries and smeared funeral ashes on his forehead. Daksha cursed Shiva. To get back at her father, Sati burned herself in the pyre of yoga. Shiva got pissed and cut off Daksha's head —notice a theme?—later replacing it with a goat, much as he had switched out his son Ganesha's head with a baby elephant many moons before. Sati was written down in legend as what a proper woman would do for her man: the practice of *suttee*, throwing yourself into the funeral pyre after your husband dies. Continuing the theme of women at the service of men, the dawn of Tantra included few feminist impulses.

Enter Durga. An evolution of the goddess Chandika, the gods crafted this seductive murderess to slay Mahisha. The god had fallen in love with her beauty. After he proposed marriage, she said she wanted to kill him, not marry him. (Score one for honesty.) To rectify any notion that women were becoming more powerful, the writer of this myth decided Durga had the 'nature' of a man but was put in a female body specifically to commit this act. Instead of being frightened, Mahisha was turned on. A counselor told him that Durga was using frightening speech to indirectly speak of her love for him. Sadly, men continue to make this error all the time. George Will's buffoonery regarding college attacks admits this: guys like to believe women say the opposite of what they mean. Mahisha wasn't as lucky as the star jock getting away with it. Durga laughed when he claimed that he was a man who makes women happy. Then she cut off his head. Surprised?

Underlying this myth is one of the key elements of the emerging Tantra: battle and intercourse are two paths of achieving unity. While both symbolize a ritual death leading to transformation, the discussion over whether or not many of these acts were actually played out or just metaphorical tales representing a person's inner state is up for debate. Most likely, both. We might shrink in horror at the idea of eating our dinner from a human skull or drinking the manna of menstrual blood combined with semen, but sects like the Aghoras were known for doing such things as both symbolic and literal ways of honoring the rites of their tradition.

Proponents of modern Tantra claim it's all about meditation, and in some respects it always was. Taking a cue from their yogi forebears, meditation was one means of raising the sacred Kundalini energy at the base of the spine to achieve union with the universe. But so was sex. Indian medical texts not only claim that male semen accomplishes this goal when 'drawn up' the spine while plunged inside a woman, they even state women too had an inner semen.

Tantric yogis were responding to the incessant pervasiveness of Brahmins, a sect that believed they were human interlopers of divine energy. Only these priests were allowed to translate mystical texts of stars and deities. Yogis felt otherwise; their rites were radicalized takes on preexisting norms. Perhaps most notable was the ritualistic practice of the Five M's: *madya* (wine), *matsya* (fish), *mamsa* (meat), *mudra* (farina, not the hand symbols in this context) and *maithuna* (sex). The conventions of purity, so essential to keeping castes in line, dissolved when Tantric yogis began ingesting these foods and using sex not as merely a procreative tool, but creatively enjoying the ecstasy it offers. In this lifestyle, both meditation (*jnana*) and action (karma) lived together harmoniously: the act and the metaphor of the action, internalized knowing and physical experience.

There is no singular path. Meditators might have been terrified by their kin drinking ungodly concoctions, yet the Aghoras would have been equally confused by Tantrikas sitting in silence imagining such acts without actually partaking in them. On one side, savages; on the other, hypocrites paying lip service to something they've never experienced. Sex has long befuddled and bewitched us. The best of intentions are transformed into the worst circumstances.

We might be able to bounce messages into space to our friend on the other side of the planet, but our brains are quite similar to these ancestors coming down from mountains into urban valleys thousands of years ago. It's not surprising these ancient ideas resonate with us today. Proto-Tantra fanatics were not the only ones to weave together violence and sex. We continue this trend today.

HUMAN BEINGS ARE WIRED to desire emotional, intellectual and physical stimuli. We need stimulation to feel alive. Being aroused feels pleasurable. There is no coincidence words like pump, arouse, and stimulation invokes images of anger and sex. Sex researchers from the Kinsey team discovered only four respects in which the physiology of anger differs from sexual arousal. Similarities are much more pronounced: each creates an increase in heart rate, pulse, blood pressure, muscular tension and breathing rate.

We appreciate sexual arousal—some are addicted to the rush of chemicals in our brains—although for the most part avoid the excitement of anger. Yet an innate drive within us craves arousal. If a human being does not have a way to express these powerful feelings, or the ability to tether these feelings to a meditation or postural practice, he defaults to this most basic of human urges. The close biological association between rage and sex is why humans have merged the two for eons. This doesn't make it ethically right; it merely helps to explain why the 'rush' of both violence and physical intimacy are acted out in similar manners, sometimes simultaneously. To men like the Indian politicians above, this feels 'natural.' In truth it is an undisciplined approach to the stark reality of our chemistry.

The word 'discipline' is important. Left to our impulses, the world is not a safe place. Ethics serve a role in keeping societies functional and healthy. The twentieth century provided positive upheaval in America. We entered and left a completely different nation. On the way in women and African-Americans (and most other foreigners) were not considered fully human. By the end not only had we made massive strides forward in equality, but set the stage for emerging activism in gay and animal rights.

Because ethical decisions are made by consensus (in a democracy, at least), we learn not only how we are built, but what needs to change. Hence, discipline. Nowhere has this been more necessary than in the eternal dance between men and women, with physical and emotional abuse and rape at the extreme end of the spectrum, though one still visited too often.

The longstanding association between violence and sex triggers our amygdala, almond-shaped groups of nuclei that process emotional reactions, help to retain memories and play a role in decision-making. Interestingly, this region works differently in men and women. One study showed that on average, women retain stronger memories after emotionally intensive events than men. The right amygdala appears to be linked to taking action after experiencing negative emotions; this side is more active in men, which helps explain the linking of trauma and violence. The left side is more passive and thoughtful, activated more often in women.

All human beings pursue avenues necessary for survival, however. Jaak Panksepp attributes this evolutionary drive to our brain's SEEKING system. When we are on the hunt, our amygdala is activated, hence the association with pleasure and reward, or seeking and satiation, propelling us forward. We hunt for food in the same manner as sex. After coupling is finished, just as after we eat a filling meal, activity in our amygdala diminishes. The pursuit is over.

Simultaneously, neural activity increases in the lateral orbitofrontal cortex (OFC) after satisfying sex and food. We are less likely to act impulsively. Our yearnings met, we no longer crave. People who have damaged their OFC show no inhibitions toward sex, sated or not. In extreme cases, they'll reach out and grab the private parts of strangers in the most inappropriate settings.

Pain and pleasure are neurologically related as well, another link in the sex/violence parallel. Women have much higher pain thresholds when sexually stimulated due to their role in childbirth. Their threshold for pain increases 40% when aroused, 100% during orgasm. Two brain regions involved in feeling pain—the insula and anterior cingulate—are both active during sexual pleasure. Professor of Neurology Anjan Chatterjee attributes this to the need for procreation: if a woman is to bear the pain of giving birth, the same networks are coopted to provide pleasure. As he writes, "An adaptive mechanism that evolved for procreation got co-opted for recreation."

This research does not bode well for the archaic fascination with celibacy. It is simply not healthy. Take Mahatma Gandhi. One of the most quoted men in the world, he was not without his dark side. Beginning in the late thirties, he required female attendants to sleep next to him on his bedroll to prove his power as a *brahmachari*. After having experimented with extreme food rations, he was applying his self-purification exercises to sex. These women had no choice in the matter. If he began shaking from the seduction of having a young female next to him, they would have to hold him with their entire body to calm him down—an odd measure, considering this would increase desire, not dampen it.

Gandhi began his own practice of *brahmacharya* in 1906 and was often unsuccessful. At his ashram he forced young boys and girls to sleep and bathe together, yet if they spoke of sex they would be punished. He bathed with his attractive personal physician; whatever attendants he forced to sleep next to him were forbidden to sleep beside their own husbands. In 1946 Gandhi began forcing his teenage grandniece, Manu, to sleep naked next to him, at times cuddling him to prove his powers. As with the other women, she had no say in the matter. Being seen and treated as a guru, he had the power to decide who did what for what purpose, so long as it fulfilled his own spiritual path. Their paths seemed irrelevant to him.

This does not discredit all the incredible work the man did or the inspirational mark he left on the world. But it does call into question the idea of a transcendent human. At this point it is necessary to call bullshit on any person who says their consciousness is on 'another plane,' and therefore material wealth and sexuality no longer affects them. While we do not yet understand the exact mechanisms of consciousness (though we are getting closer), physiology exposes the lies in such sentiments. It becomes all about the leader, never the followers. Gandhi's case highlights this: the psychological and emotional trauma suffered by his female servants is one facet history has abandoned. Before and after his time many other 'enlightened' men have made the same claims, to the same disastrous results.

Consider a yogi who rose above chauvinism. Tirumalai Krishnamacharya is the man most responsible for bringing yoga to the world, instructing B.K.S. Iyengar and Pattabhi Jois, among many others. He was challenged by India's social norms and women on a number of occasions. While he first refused to change his mind, he slowly expanded it, with incredible results.

Indra Devi is one example. Born in Latvia as Zhenia Labunskaia, this young woman disputed Krishnamacharya when asking him to be her teacher: she was female *and* a foreigner. He balked. She persisted. Finally he gave in, prescribing her a tormenting schedule and intense dietary restrictions. The Ayurveda master figured she would fold. Instead, within a year of her apprenticeship, Devi endeared Krishnamacharya. They became lifelong friends. Her 1953 book, *Forever Young, Forever Healthy*, was an international bestseller. She lived to be 102 years old, and her schools remain open in Buenos Aires, Argentina, where she became something of a local saint. Her Sai Yoga, which includes chanting and prayer, influences other styles today. Krishnamacharya had previously avoided mantras. Because of Devi's influence he incorporated them into his teachings.

Then there was his son, T.K.V. Desikachar. Krishnamacharya would tie him up in postures and leave him there for hours, which increased Desikachar's loathing of yoga. Another encounter with a female again altered an attitude. Having graduated with a degree in engineering, Desikachar watched as his father was approached by a European woman who jumped out of her car to hug him. For a *brahman* to be embraced by a woman in public was taboo. Desikachar asked his father about it. He replied that the woman hadn't been able to sleep without the assistance of drugs for twenty years. Thanks to his yoga prescription, she was now drug-free. An epiphany struck Desikachar; he begged his father for instruction. Abandoning a career in engineering, this apprenticeship lasted twenty-eight years. Desikachar applied his father's knowledge in the Vinyasa system known as Viniyoga, practiced worldwide though virtually unknown in America.

Two influential yoga practices developed from Krishnamacharya's ability to look beyond the conventions of his culture and offer practices for everyone. Then in 2012, the great yogi's grandson Kausthub left his position at the Krishnamacharya Healing and Yoga Foundation in Chennai after allegations of sexual misconduct and verbal and emotional abuse of female students arose. Two steps forward, another back.

TANTRA BROUGHT US INTO our bodies. Many older strains of yoga were all about escaping the flesh. The slow transformation of yoga into Tantra discovered the body as a vehicle for self-transformation. But transformation into what?

I personally get lost in the literature when tales of levitation, psychic powers and 'diamond bodies' emerge. Hallucinations are as old as human beings. One theory of yoga's origins links it to the miracle drug of the archaic age: soma. This hallucinogenic juice was revered in the Vedas. Research shows it was most likely a tea brewed of psychedelic mushrooms, the strain *Amanita muscaria*. One hymn to soma goes like this:

We have drunk the soma / we have become immortal / we have gone to the light / we have found the gods / What can hatred and the malice of a mortal do to us now? / The glorious drops that I have drunk set me free in wide space.

Sounds like a good trip to me.

Soma hymns disappeared from the literature as Indians climbed down from mountains, where mushrooms were in abundance, to newly forming cities, where they were not. Suddenly the same metaphors—flight, wide-open spaces, mingling with deities—were being accomplished through breathing techniques like Breath of Fire and Kapalbhati. This has led some scholars to wonder whether yoga was created due to entheogenic cosmonauts seeking a fix. That would be one startling revelation: yoga's origins in psychedelia.

While celebration of the body is a good thing, distortions through sexual and emotional abuse have been rampant for millennia. If transformation is accomplished at the expense of another what good comes from it? Assigning sex with poetic flourishes and as a means of deepening personal bonds with a partner is a beautiful reshaping of this biological impulse. We seem nowhere near able to shed the practice of its shadow, however.

Which is why *brahmacharya* is the most flawed *yama*. The metaphors of Patanjali no longer serve us: sacred semen only applies to one-half of the population. In a country where yoginis well outnumber yogis, it doesn't work. We can sit here for years and deconstruct numerous prohibitions against sex throughout the ages. Tantra, for one, was driven underground in India after the British began enforcing Victorian codes of conduct, something that certainly did not advance the psyche of the patriarch.

America has its own battles thanks to Puritanism. Cultural shifts in marriage have shocked the notion of traditional unions. The plight against same-sex couples waged by members of religious sects stems from an inability to hold up a mirror and look at the nuclear family, a term practically incinerated. Divorce rates are at an all-time high while happiness in relationships is nose-diving. Forget about online dating sites catering to single adults looking for love: Tinder, an app no deeper than looks and hook-ups had over ten million daily users in April 2014, while services like Ashley Madison specifically target married individuals looking for other married folk. The company's tagline is 'Life is short. Have an affair.' Twenty-one million people have signed up worldwide.

Studying human sexuality is especially daunting given the nature of research. It's hard to become aroused if you're in an fMRI machine or trying to get it on with scientists watching. Not so for rats. Researchers inserting catheters into rodent brains found that a male rat's nucleus accumbens was flooded with dopamine when separated from a female rat. Once the barrier is opened and the male gets what he wants, levels of the hormone drop sharply. Show him another female and dopamine surges again. Rats are used in labs because their DNA is not far from that of humans. I'm sure many women would agree the terms 'sex' and 'rodents' go together.

A new ethos emerging from our sexual proclivities might save some marriages, even if they don't look like our grandparents' households. Therapist Esther Perel, dubbed a 'sexual healer' by the *NY Times*, has extensively researched the benefits of affairs. On this topic she writes, "Very often we don't go elsewhere because we are looking for another person. We go elsewhere because we are looking for another self. It isn't so much that we want to leave the person we are with as we want to leave the person we have become."

A powerful insight into the fragmented nature of identity. In my life I've cheated and been cheated on. Neither has left me fulfilled. The best relationships I've been in were the most honest. This dance is never easy. There is precedent: researchers have found that basic kindnesses expressed by couples were key to sustaining a relationship. Psychologist John Gottman and his colleague Robert Levonson divided the couples he spent decades researching into 'masters' and 'disasters.' When a man called his wife over to look at a bird outside of the window, her response made a huge difference in the longevity of their marriage. A master expresses interest and goes over, even if she doesn't really care about birds. The disaster checks her phone while telling him to leave her alone.

The sacrifice of relationship plays out in such small acts. Sex is an intimate act tough for some to open up to. We are vulnerable creatures. When inhuman demands regarding restrictions and morality are placed upon us, layers of anxiety mask true connection, to our partners, to ourselves. Unbridled honesty is a daunting prospect, but worth it. Anything less leads to the myriad distortions we've investigated over these pages.

Yoga is a series of techniques designed to transform the self. Ethics and morals provide a doorway to step through and begin an internal investigation. I for one have no desire to pull the metaphorical Kundalini up my chakras, or any of the other promises of Tantra or Patanjali. An honest relationship with myself and the people I share my life with is way more spiritual than sitting alone thinking the universe is observing me meditate, or using the term spirituality to engage with my carnal desires.

On how to build this relationship with ourselves, sometimes old advice is good advice. The *Shata Patha Brāhmana* states it best: one becomes that which one contemplates. Let us now investigate the effort this requires.

6 TAPAS : PUMP UP THE VOLUME

WENDELL POTTER HAD HIS Buddha moment.

As the top publicity executive for health insurer CIGNA, Potter was on the job on July 18, 2007, when he decided to visit a health fair in Wise County, Virginia. It might have been chance that he was visiting his parents in Tennessee, but his duties involved tailing political contenders who advocated for widespread health care. With presidential hopeful John Edwards speaking, Potter hopped in his father's car and drove northeast.

Potter grew up in rural Tennessee. Winding roads through rural pastures were not new to him. After college he patrolled his state's beat as a political and business reporter until a career in public relations offered more money and prestige. Initially joining the team at Baptist Health System of East Tennessee, he worked his way up the corporate ladder, first to Humana, Inc., then to CIGNA, one of the nation's largest for-profit health care providers. His job mainly entailed writing spin pieces for the press and inventing language to protect the interests of his employer. He led the charge in discrediting Michael Moore when he released *Sicko* and penned much of the fear-mongering language around President Barack Obama's initiatives. Potter was an early tagline man for Tea Party placards, the spinster who invented nightmares where none existed.

Thus he arrived in Virginia to dream up new spin to combat Edwards. The CIGNA CEO loathed the North Carolina Senator's talk of broad health care coverage and industry reforms. Instead of focusing on Edwards' messaging, however, Potter wandered around clinic grounds. People had tented overnight just to get a good place in line. When he passed through the gates, a revelation struck.

"The scene inside was surreal. Hundreds of people, many of them soaking wet from the rain that had been falling all morning, were waiting in lines that stretched out of view. As I walked around, I noticed that some of those lines led to barns and cinder block buildings with row after row of animal stalls, where doctors and nurses were treating patients… Except for curtains serving as makeshift doors on the animal stalls, there was little privacy. And unlike health fairs I had seen in shopping centers and malls, this was a real clinic. Dentists were pulling teeth and filling cavities, optometrists were examining eyes for glaucoma and cataracts, doctors and nurses were doing Pap smears and mammograms, surgeons were cutting out skin cancers, and gastroenterologists were conducting sigmoidoscopies."

Rewind roughly two millennia. Siddhatta Gotama's father had tried to shield his son from the world's miseries. A rich and respected elder in Kapilavatthu, he had done his best to ensure an easy life for the young prince. Yet there was nothing rewarding about being pent up in an estate or his path of marriage and fatherhood. At age twenty-nine, a few days after the birth of his son, Rāhula (which means 'fetter,' for the Buddha felt the boy would shackle him), Gotama began his epic journey of asceticism, meditation and the philosophy bearing his name today. His father spent years keeping him imprisoned inside of his home until the future Buddha demanded a tour of the surrounding village. As the mythology goes, he witnessed the realities of aging, illness, corruption, sorrow and death. Once exposed to these mortal truths, he refused to live in confinement when most people experienced an entirely different reality. He had to make a difference, luxury be damned.

Which is exactly the revelation Wendell Potter had while walking around the clinic that cloudy summer day. He was witnessing the consequences of his job in real time, those sick and dying Americans who could not afford coverage. In his book Potter mentions that roughly 45,000 Americans die every year because they lack health insurance. He admits his responsibility in helping boost that statistic. It is both a confession and declaration. His duties at CIGNA lost all meaning. Potter realized he was a major player in a system that was not providing health, but death, all for the bottom line of executives and shareholders. Not only did he quit his high paying six-figure job, he has devoted his life to exposing the deceptive reality of the industry he spent so much of life helping create.

In June, 2009, Potter stood before the US Senate Commerce, Science and Transportation Committee to deliver testimony regarding the inner workings of the insurance industry. He freely offered the spin techniques devised to keep Americans uninsured and underinsured to satisfy Wall Street investors. He now lectures on the topic and writes for progressive publications and websites, himself a leading proponent of universal health care. He has taken the poison of the world, much like the blue-throated Shiva, Nīlakaṇtha, who drank the toxic ocean and transformed it so humanity could survive. Mythologies are accolades to human feats. In this, Potter's remaking has a long precedence of people who have had a change of heart and decided, despite personal fortune, to make the planet a better place.

TAPAS ARE NOT ONLY the appetizers you receive for free with each drink in Spain. In yoga philosophy, *tapas* means 'heat' or 'glow.' Initially developed by ascetics wanting to get out of their head and body through intense, repetitive breathing exercises, *tapas* can be equally destructive if misused. For example, people suffering from anxiety disorder should not practice Breath of Fire, Kapalbhati, or Bellows Breath, as they can trigger sensitive nervous systems. As the *Tattva Vaisharadi* notes, *tapas* should not upset the body's physiological balance. If it becomes torturous or emaciates the body, it is destructive, antithetical to treating the temple respectfully— although some scriptures, such as the *Yoga Yajnavalkya*, endorse such treatment. From a modern perspective of physical and mental health, extreme asceticism is a hindrance.

The *Bhagavad Gītā* considers ascetic practices selfish. If you are so concerned with the 'blowing out' of your brain and body, there is no concern of your duty to the tribe. We experience toned down versions today, when students leave class early without putting their props away or cleaning up after themselves. They've had their workout; someone else can clean up after them. This mentality is sadly pervasive. I notice this in the bathroom when men leave the faucet running while shaving or, worse, walk away with the tap on and leave their towels on the ground. This is, of course, a different form of selfishness, although it still demands more work of others, so is similar at the foundation.

Such seemingly minor selfish patterns certainly do not equate to the total bodily and emotional purification goals of early yogis. Yet if we do not notice small everyday habits informing the larger perspective of our personality, we miss the point. Having someone else clean up after our mess requires a privileged attitude. If purification is our target, small tasks are the arrows we aim with. According to the *Gītā*, three different practices comprise *tapas*: bodily, vocal and mental austerities. Let's consider them one by one.

IF YOU PRACTICE YOGA, you've probably been in a class in which the instructor notes the 5,000-year-old lineage of yoga. This is a loose interpretation. If they are referring to the process one goes through trying to explain their place in the world, sure, yoga's likely older. But if your teacher was referencing the series of postures you've been flowing through, nothing could be further from the truth.

Classical references to *asanas* do exist. Standing on one's head, for example, dates back to at least the *Yogatattva Upanisad*. Later Hatha Yoga texts started adding poses as the years progressed. Postures do not seem confined to yoga manuals, though. Professor of Anthropology Joseph S. Alter found *sirsasana* in the sixteenth century text, *Mallapurana*, as an exercise program for medieval wrestlers. Alter discovered no examples of the beloved *surya namaskar*—sun salutation, the essential building block of modern Hatha-Vinyasa yoga—anywhere before the nineteenth century. Most of what we call yoga today was created in west central India in the second decade of the twentieth century, many of the postures not more than a few decades old.

The reason for the re-creation of yoga is simple enough: pride. While the British Raj officially ruled India from 1858-1947, it had maintained a presence in the country for centuries. Trade routes were governed by national agencies, extracting silks and spices from India to set off fashion trends in Europe. The British felt that Indians cut a submissive culture and acted accordingly. By the dawn of the twentieth century, weightlifting and wrestling became a way for Indians to express dignity. Physical image offered mental clarity. By bulking up, they would eventually ward off their oppressor with might. The few postures known in yoga were considered effeminate. Sitting around meditating was not going to build the army they needed. Physicality trumped introspection. Yogis had to adjust.

Recently there has been much chatter online about the validity of the 'yoga selfie,' yogis and yoginis posting daily photos in challenging postures. Fans claim it inspires people; detractors say it is egotistical and self-serving. This trend, however, is not new. At the turn of the twentieth century yogis showboated poses in public displays of athleticism, much in the way that body builders flex for the camera (or women passing by). Yogis were also master salesmen, reading palms, selling magical charms, and interpreting dreams for the paying customer. Then, as now, critics saw this emphasis on postures as a bastardization of the discipline. Yogis were emphasizing only one limb of Patanjali's eightfold prescription. The cult of the body was winning out.

What has emerged from this glorification of the physical is paradoxical. Yogis claim that the postures are gateways to self-knowledge and higher consciousness, creating a spiritual connection that regular exercise cannot provide. The postures themselves, not the benefits of meditation or *pranayama*, have supplanted the other seven limbs. We've gone from trying to escape the body to worshipping it on our smart phone.

It's hard to buy into the idea that yoga poses are particularly special. One can get the same high from dance and martial arts, interval training and cardiovascular exercise. The only truly different components of yoga are an emphasis on breathing, meditation and relaxation. In fact, the majority of clinically studied health benefits deal with this softer side: the concentration attained during focused (and even nondirective) meditation, the physiological bonus you receive from *savasana* and the wonderful effects of restorative postures on your nervous system.

While yoga is sometimes touted as a weight loss wonder and heart-healthy necessity, the science has not held up. Chances are you will not lose weight because yoga *slows* your metabolism. To be clear, the body awareness sometimes coinciding with yoga might help you create better lifestyle and dietary choices, which subsequently helps shed pounds. Even rigorous forms of yoga, such as Ashtanga, do not provide the cardiovascular and fat burning benefits of running and interval training. Yoga is designed to slow things down, not speed things up, irrespective of how many suns you salute.

I'm not criticizing yoga as an exercise format. Quite the opposite. I don't treat a student any differently whether they're trying to get in touch with their inner selves or tone their arms and legs. Criticizing yoga's physicality misses an important point: human beings are built to move. The sedentary lifestyle Americans now specialize in is tragic, a damaging pattern that has caused skyrocketing obesity rates. We need to move.

The different ways of achieving a balanced chemical and hormonal state depends on individual preferences. *How* we get there is not as important as *that* we get there. Sadly, physical exercise is at least partly economic. A significant population cannot afford to spend hours every week working out. Like many other aspects of our society, there are tiers depending on one's financial situation. This sadly has consequences on our national health.

Let's briefly investigate the younger generation and how this trend starts. Our culture has slowly eroded the two most important means of achieving a mind-body connection in public schools. At a time when science is proving the significant impact movement and artistic endeavors have had on our evolution, American legislators and school officials are cleansing the national educational system of music and arts programs and physical education classes. Harboring a shortsighted focus on science and technology—important, though only two pieces of an interlocking puzzle—these officials are abandoning crucial aspects of learning in favor of what they feel necessary to compete on a global scale. Unsurprisingly institutions that fail to offer the arts and physical education often perform lowest in the subjects educators are so desperately trying to improve. The result is a strange pivot toward what are considered relevant academic subjects without a proper understanding of the creative and physical underpinnings needed for optimizing our learning process. Mind/body is not an either/or. It's two ways of looking at one animal.

According to a 2012 report by the Center on Budget and Priority Policies, more than 95% of children attending school have seen a budget decrease since the recession. With a growing emphasis on academia, educators are missing a stark reality: low-income high school students who compiled no arts credits in four years are five times less likely to graduate than students in the same income bracket who study the arts.

Performing music together, for example, is an important social bonding skill during a time of awkward growing pains. It also releases endorphins, similar to the euphoric 'runner's high,' which has been shown to promote feelings of wellbeing and relaxation—both important qualities to cultivate if you want to retain information. More generally, listening to music elevates mood, increases endurance, reduces perceived effort, and may even help promote metabolic efficiency. Hearing music you enjoy affects your supplementary motor area, basal ganglia, ventral premotor cortex, and cerebellum, all of which help coordination. Background music has been proven to help surgeons increase alertness and concentration, both important skills in their line of duty, yet also key in helping keep students' attention while in class.

Interestingly, our brain is the only place in the world that music exists. That singular organ has the ability to translate seemingly disparate noises from a range of sources and mix them together into what we call music. Nothing affects so many regions of our brain as music, yet it has no singular music center. As a symphony orchestra begins to play and new instruments are introduced, different regions of our brain are activated. In fact, just thinking about a song fires the same neurons as if you were actually listening it.

The same is true for movement. If I tell you to envision Warrior One, the same areas of your brain will activate as if you were in the pose. But envisioning exercise is no replacement for the real thing. Harvard University Associate Clinical Professor of Psychiatry John J. Ratey believes the healthiest thing we can do for our brains is move our bodies. Proteins produced by engaging our muscles travel through our bloodstream to our brains and play important roles in our highest thought processes. As he writes, "When we exercise, particularly if the exercise requires complex motor movement, we're also exercising the areas of the brain involved in the full suite of cognitive functions."

This makes sense from an evolutionary perspective. Our ancestors didn't need to coin a special term for exercise as their daily lives included plenty of physical labor. Post-industrial societies were the first to introduce automation and specialization. As our forebears moved from farms and villages to urban environments and became more sedentary, partaking in this special thing called exercise became a necessity. Those who partook fared much better cognitively than those who sat around, as my grandmother used to say, on their *tookuses*.

A case study at Naperville Central High School near Chicago proves this point. After implementing a program called Zero Hour PE—a volunteer pre-class workout session—students opting in for the morning fitness regimen showed a 17% improvement in reading and comprehension skills. What's more, Zero Hour students taking literacy classes directly after working out increased scores more dramatically than fellow Zero classmates taking the same class at the end of the day. Ratey's prescription for studying for a test? Right after an aerobic workout. Your brain retains information better.

Colombian neuroscientist Rodolfo R. Llinás believes thinking is the "evolutionary internalization of movement." Just as our brain produces thoughts, a certain form of movement within our minds, our body is designed to move. It makes sense that we excel in our highest cognitive endeavors, and by extension understand and control our entire emotional landscape, when we exercise. The old yogis knew physicality was important when including bodily austerities in their doctrine of *tapas*. Whatever one believes the body is a vehicle *for*, moving it is a must. Yoga is one wonderful method among many. None should be thought of as 'lesser.' As long as we're moving, the physiological paycheck is worthwhile. The mental and emotional clarity that follows exercise is an essential building block in creating a strong society.

"A PRACTICE LIKE CHANTING has a number of different ways that it allows the mind to settle, rather than grabbing it and holding it down. Purification is a really powerful word, and it shouldn't be thought of as meaning pure and impure, good and bad. All this attachment we have for stuff and for who we think we are, what we want and don't want, there's a certain amount of energy that's frustrated within us because we don't know how to get what we want. So you're never going to be able to calm your mind with that energy because all that energy wants to do is get off."

I'm sitting in a car on 14th St and Sixth Ave with Krishna Das, America's most well-known *kirtan* singer, interviewing him for my 2005 book, *Global Beat Fusion*. KD has kindly offered me a ride after a performance at Dharma Yoga Center, and we were discussing the benefits of his craft. While I haven't chanted often, the few times I've attended a *kirtan* I've felt the sort of clarity he mentions. Our brains love repetition; chanting serves this function. By expressing a series of Sanskrit syllables over and over within a community, Americans have recreated this ancient Indian tradition, akin to the African-Americans who made gospel come alive for centuries. Singing in a ritualistic context is powerful medicine.

Playing music together is one of humanity's oldest rituals. The late English psychiatrist Anthony Storr writes that music's primary function is collective and communal. "People sing together, dance together, in every culture, and one can imagine them doing so, around the first fires, a hundred thousand years ago." In fact, some neuroscientists believe the vocalizations involved in singing was an ancestral attempt of expressing emotions, and may have led to the eventual appearance of language.

Yogis I know attend *kirtans* for the experience of chanting with like-minded people. The emotions we feel when we listen to music are reflected in our brain. Not only are the higher areas of the brain activated, each and every limbic and paralimbic brain structure can be affected. According to Dan Levitin, our brains release emotionally-charged neurochemicals such as dopamine, prolactin, and the 'trust hormone' oxytocin that fosters, for one, the all-important bond between mother and infant.

When we identify with music's expressive aspects, awakened by the emotions it conveys, we experience music empathetically. When our emotions are provoked by music, our brain matches the emotional state of what we're hearing. This involves two separate processes: a cognitive process (where we comprehend the feelings of what the music is conveying) and the emotional aspect (feeling what the music is expressing). Within music there's an opportunity to distinguish between our individuality and another human being. In this sense music is the 'other.' We identify with this other and understand its situation, feelings, and motives, moving us beyond mere altruism toward true compassion for other human beings.

Music kindles emotions using the same neuronal mechanisms as when we understand other people's affective states. This is occurring in the brainstem, hypothalamus, and amygdala, the neural mechanisms underlying empathy and caring. According to Levitin, music serves an evolutionary purpose and is also a natural phenomenological expression of human spirituality. He believes it replicates the ability for humans to care, trust, love, and be deeply moved by something. Oxytocin released in the brains of people playing music together is unifying, the reason why yogis chanting mantras feel connected to one another.

The 'cleansing' aspects of vocal austerities are derived from the flooding of our brain with pleasure-inducing hormones. This is the payment from our brain's pleasure/reward system, partaking in an artistic expression that is very likely our oldest known form of communication. It makes me recall an old Zimbabwean saying: *If you can walk you can dance / If you can talk you can sing.* While hard to imagine today, for most of history thousands of songs could not be carried in your pocket. You had to actually play an instrument and sing, or at the very least attend a performance. We were once all active participants in the process of music.

Sometimes *tapas* is presented as a rigorous discipline. If you are practicing breath-altering *kriyas* this is certainly the case. But not all work has to be hard. This is the elegance of evolution: life can be pleasurable. Vocal austerities also include how we use language, such as not gossiping or talking negatively about others. In terms of singing, though, we know it does a brain good, in the shower and well beyond.

PURUSHA IS THE TERM denoting the transcendental self. Man must travel through the illusory wormhole that is *prakriti*—the word is defined as 'creatrix,' so *Matrix* symbolism is appropriate—to spill into the universal awareness known as *purusha*. It is man outside of man, man beyond man, a soul somehow inside and outside, nowhere and everywhere simultaneously. Whatever the 'true' origins of yoga, there is little argument that detangling *purusha* from *prakriti* was the ultimate goal: the psychedelic brain states one attains from the *kriyas*, the deeply reflective inner peace after meditation. *Samadhi* is the state one achieves when the *purusha* is finally detached, the witness of existence peering inside the witnessing human being.

In writing the *Yoga Sutras*, Patanjali was more a compiler than an innovator. He recorded an emerging synthesis of techniques designed to yank *purusha* from the rest of creation. This yoga was very different from what we practice today. As religious historian Karen Armstrong writes, "Yoga was a systematic assault on the ego, an exacting regimen that over a long period of time taught the aspirant to abolish his normal consciousness with its errors and delusions, and replace it with the ecstatic discovery of his *purusha*."

Attaining a transcendent state has little to do with our conception of divinity. These yogis, taking clues from early Sāmkhya teachings, were atheistic. There was nothing supernatural about their practices. Yoga was focused entirely on developing human potential to the fullest. It was an introspective experience, a springboard into higher consciousness. Not until the *bhakti* movement was the role of gods an integral component in yoga, and even then deities were not treated as external agents but as internal mechanisms for shifting consciousness. They were malleable because they mimicked the humans they were created to represent.

Gotama became aware of this confusion between divinities and humans during his training in yoga. After leaving his palace he wandered into the city of Vesāli to study under a local Sāmkhya instructor named Alāra Kālāma. Sāmkhya means 'discrimination,' and would play an important role in the later development of Buddhism. There Gotama was trained in the cultivation of his intellect in an attempt to separate *purusha* from *prakriti* by using sheer mental force. Gotama quickly ascended the ranks, with a promise by Kālāma that he would soon embody these teachings by 'direct knowledge' in the lineage from teacher to student. This did not sit well with Gotama, who felt that no human being could offer such an awakening. Liberation, or nirvana, could not be transferred from another or descend supernaturally from some foreign energy. It could only come by discipline and dedication, one of the hallmarks in the philosophy he would go on to create. Buddha was always anti-guru.

It is not uncommon to find Buddhism and yoga entwined today. Buddha statues are common in yoga studios around the world. Of course, the young sage named Gotama was anything but a deity. He would have said that he was a human being exploiting his brain's capacity for freeing itself from the shackles of bondage. That bondage, he knew, came from his own thought patterns. He would come, in his own way, to embrace the three aspects of *tapas* mentioned in this chapter: the bodily austerities in asceticism, ultimately choosing a balanced lifestyle as the best way to cultivate a focused and calm mind; the vocal austerities in his Eightfold Noble Path, in which Right Speech is a crucial component; and finally the mental austerities in his practice of meditation. In regards to our job here in this book, that last one is of special importance and deserves its own chapter. The purifying technique of meditation as represented in the discipline of *tapas* gets you in your seat. What happens there begins the next *niyama*: the realm of self-study.

7 SVADHYAYA : TURNING THE MIRROR

TWO MONKS ARE WALKING. They approach a river when spotting a woman who is having trouble crossing. She sees the monks and runs over to plead for help. One monk turns his head. The other kneels down, tells her to climb onto his back and carries her across. When they have reached the other side, she thanks him and the two friends continue on their journey.

After a few miles of silence, one monk is infuriated. Unable to hold back his anger any longer, he turns to the other. "We're monks. You know we're not allowed to talk to women, much less touch them. How could you betray the order like that?"

The other monk, calm as ever, replies, "I put her down at the riverbank. Why are you still carrying her?"

STORIES SUCH AS THIS comprise one aspect of *svādhyāya*, or 'study one's own (*sva*) going into (*adhyāya*).' The monk chose service over the rigidity of his order, something his friend was unable to grasp. This *niyama* is designed for the investigation of your entire being. Initially it was dreamt up as a study aid for those learning the Vedas. It was thought that through the repetition of sacred texts the adept would be able to transcend his personal identity by connecting with his *purusha*. The spiritual power gained through this process puts one at ease and cultivates a sense of peace.

The writer of the *Vishnu Purāna* considers *svādhyāya* a perfect complement to yoga: "From study one should proceed to Yoga and from Yoga to study. Through perfection in study and Yoga, the supreme Self becomes manifest. Study is one eye with which to behold that [Self], and Yoga is the other."

This study doesn't only occur on your meditation cushion. Recognizing your mental patterns is an important step; your actions become a testament to your humanity. For example, you might realize that developing empathy and cultivating presence is important. You post quotes by the Dalai Lama and Pema Chödrön on Twitter. But then later that day you talk on the phone while purchasing something as if the cashier was not even there, a mere inconvenience to your end of making a purchase. Where did those qualities go? Is the cashier an inhuman cog? How do we close this distance between intention and action?

Meditation is one answer. Neuroscience has shown that its benefits extend well beyond the cushion. Before we get there, let's see what our brain is actually doing by investigating exactly what this thing we're yoking to in yoga is all about.

MOST OF OUR UNDERSTANDING of the human brain comes from trauma. This started with a famous incident involving Phineas Gage, a nineteenth century railroad construction foreman. On September 13, 1848, Gage was working in Vermont when an iron rod shot out from a hole into his left eye clean through the other side of his head, landing some eighty feet away. Miraculously he survived. While there are conflicting accounts as to how this changed his behavior, his friends no longer recognized the man they once knew as Phineas. His entire demeanor dramatically shifted. An important medical breakthrough followed when doctors realized that the brain's functions are localized. Different regions affected not only different parts of Gage's body, but his interior world of feelings and thoughts. This knowledge greatly expanded our understanding of the human brain. We realized we don't have a fixed identity. Chemistry plays a pivotal role. And that chemistry can change us, either consciously or through trauma, in what has been termed neuroplasticity.

The notion of a predetermined human being fit old religious models. If we were created in God's image, or if our soul was born into a certain caste, a divine reason must have existed. The best we could do is whatever we accomplished with our limited gifts—unless of course we were a prince, or a *brahman*, or born to a billionaire, in which case the blessings bestowed upon us were thanks to beatific favor. The Buddha's case alone should be explanation enough for the plasticity of the brain. His dismissal of luxury for monastic robes was certainly dramatic. Yet it took science time to catch up. If Gotama were alive today, he'd be a neuroscientist.

Since Gage's accident, doctors have turned to trauma victims to investigate how our brains operate. Exceptions often aid us in discovering how norms function. Granted, neuroscience is not a perfect field. The ability to actually monitor and record through noninvasive fMRI technology is only a few decades old, an infant at best. When we discuss emotions connected to neural regions, we're looking at what area is activated when correlated to specific thoughts and visual or auditory aids. It's rare that one specific region is ever completely responsible for any single emotion or action. Like the Buddhist idea of interdependence, our brain is comprised of many regions of one organ, just as many members make up one *sangha*. Still, the current model is an evolutionary step up from needing to slice skulls open, and we're quickly learning as new technologies emerge.

The road to neuroplasticity was not easy. For centuries our brain had been treated like a machine. This metaphor persists when our brain is referenced as a computer, as if memory was something simply stored in folders, or when we think vision is like the tiny eye of a camera on top of our laptops, staring out to snap shots of reality. Our visual system is actually comprised of thirty different regions, each specialized in one aspect of sight, such as depth, color and focus. Damage to any one of those radically alters how we see the world.

The science of neuroplasticity, or malleability, emerged in the sixties and seventies as scientists realized our brain changes its actual structure when different tasks are being performed. This was observed in stroke victims, who were assumed to never be able to perform old tasks. While it is true the damaged section is never used again, a diligent patient with a persistent therapist exploits under-utilized brain regions to relearn skills. Our brain is constantly adapting to learn under the circumstances, even if it requires circumnavigating areas not designed for the task.

The very notion of a self is contained in our brain, another facet of this science some have trouble accepting. Modern spirituality is filled with disembodied spirits, divine energies, and reincarnating souls in attempts of explaining perceived gaps in our experiences. In the past decade alone neuroscientists have shown that seeing auras is a form of synesthesia and out-of-body experiences can be recreated in laboratories. As journalist

Norman Doidge has written, plasticity is not only the key to cognitive flexibility, it also has the potential to increase our stubbornness by strengthening certain neural ties, what he calls the 'plastic paradox.' Think of the agnostic who nearly dies and has a religious conversion. Every bit of effort during recovery is funneled into this container of being born-again. Each experience is associated with divine favor, strengthening the bond between physical healing and spiritual assistance.

There's good reason that our brain seeks patterns. Our ancestors needed this cognitive ability for survival. If you noticed a tail sticking out from one end of a bush and an ear near the other, you knew you had to run, or at the very least, find a large rock as quickly as possible. Our brain hates gaps, so it's quite natural that we'd piece together a story with whatever information is available. During a drought you might sacrifice a goat to the sky gods. If an earthquake destroyed a neighboring village perhaps you fasted for a week to ensure the same fate wouldn't befall yours. African hunters liked to put bullets in their mouths before loading them into their guns as a way of 'tasting' the meat. There has been no end to magical thinking in our species.

Which is why it is frustrating when people claim science can't explain everything, or that it takes the magic out of life. Quite the opposite: the gelatinous organ in our head, with its 100 billion neurons each having approximately 10,000 synaptic connections to other neurons, is responsible for every mythology, every technology, every thought ever expressed, everything ever built in our world. If you believe this is anything less than miraculous, print out this beautiful passage from neuroscientist V.S. Ramachandran: "How can a three-pound mass of jelly that you can hold in your palm imagine angels, contemplate the meaning of infinity, and even question its own place in the cosmos? Especially awe inspiring is the fact that any single brain, including yours, is made up of atoms that were forged in the hearts of countless, far-flung stars billions of years ago. These particles drifted for eons and light-years until gravity and chance brought them together here, now. These atoms now form a conglomerate—your brain—that can not only ponder the very stars that gave it birth but can also think about its own ability to think and wonder about its own ability to wonder."

The brain is well equipped to wax poetic about itself with no damage to the science behind its workings. Just because consciousness retains its mysterious nature does not mean it's a riddle that cannot be solved, or that we'll lose anything by figuring out the mechanisms by which it operates. Imagine if you showed up at your doctor's office with stomach pains. He asks if you've eaten anything suspect. You reply that you haven't. Ok, he replies, he's run out of ideas, best of luck to you. Chances are you'd find a new doctor. Immediately.

Yet we treat medical researchers as if they should have all diseases figured out. We demand an immediate diagnosis. All illnesses and imbalances have a cause—a physical cause that, if not curable, can be treated in some manner. This is widely accepted. Yet we freeze when it comes to potentially figuring out the origins of consciousness. Any hint of discovering that what we've believed to be true is actually not the case shatters our perception of the universe and our role in it. Best it is to remain mysterious.

This is why Buddha, after leaving his yoga training, had his revelation: all life is *dukkha*. While normally translated as suffering, Karen Armstrong finds 'unsatisfactory' and 'flawed' to be better terms; psychotherapist Mark Epstein prefers 'hard to face.' Life is not what we want it to be. Our brain, loathing missing jigsaw puzzle pieces, invents what's absent on the spot, regardless of whether or not it has anything to with the larger picture. As Armstrong writes about spirituality, a sentiment that holds up equally well with neuroscience, "Even if the familiar is unsatisfactory, we tend to cling to it because we are afraid of the unknown."

Like the plastic paradox, awry imaginations have created everything we see around us. We might fear the unknown but the tales we've invented due to it are astounding. Our brain is a born storyteller. *Maya* is its ability to spin numerous tales, some to our benefit, others to our detriment. On average we daydream 2,000 times per day, each lasting up to fourteen seconds. As author Jonathan Gottschall figured out, we spend roughly one-third of our lives living in fantasy. If yoga is the art of staying present, it is up against the most non-present entity possible.

This is the larger picture of being human. We share the same fantastical abilities for inventing stories. What those stories are and how they're told is as different as the individual lives we lead. All of those countless synaptic connections leave a lot of room for variety. This is not to say storytelling is bad. Cultures are created through mythologies. The previously mentioned study in Norway discovered that closing your eyes and letting your brain go on a tangent has wonderful health benefits, and can positively affect those around you by feeding their imagination.

Yoga has rarely been nondirective, however. How the mind is directed has varied over the ages. That study essentially deals with mindfulness, the Buddhist practice of observing your thoughts as if you were a witness watching someone else. This is one important layer of self-study: observing the observer which is you, the brain contemplating itself. Meditation can also be directive, and through this we are empowered. It is possible to make real changes in our lives by focusing our thoughts in a direction. There is nothing mystical or magical about this. It is simply what our brains do. And it is quite amazing.

IN 1992, UNIVERSITY OF Wisconsin-Madison Professor of Psychology and Psychiatry Richard J. Davidson wrote a letter to the Dalai Lama requesting an opportunity to study expert meditators living in the hills around Dharamsala, where the venerable leader has lived in exile since 1959. Davidson himself had been meditating for years and knew the neural benefits first hand, but his colleagues were skeptical of this New Age-sounding practice. Launching a serious study into meditation's effects would have resulted in smug laughter. Davidson persevered; he wanted to understand how thousands of hours of meditation alter brain circuitry. To his surprise, he received a blessing. Tenzin Gyatso, the current Tibetan leader, has long been interested in science, and has spent a good portion of his career studying how the sciences verify and discredit Buddhist philosophy. As he writes, "If scientific analysis were conclusively to demonstrate certain claims in Buddhism to be false, then we must accept the findings of science and abandon those claims."

Davidson struggled during his initial efforts. Heavy equipment carted up treacherous mountainsides to interview unreceptive monks did not produce usable data. In the process, however, Davidson and Gyatso became friends. Eventually the researcher did scan a number of meditators, beginning with French Buddhist monk Matthieu Ricard. In 1972 Ricard nearly completed his doctoral thesis in molecular genetics before leaving a promising career in science to study Tibetan Buddhism. His willingness to meditate in a laboratory stems from his knowledge of science's potential benefits. Like Gyatso, he has been a leading figure in merging science and spirituality, provided neither is compromised in the process.

Meditation is the heart of Buddhist and yoga practice. Yogis have long known that it greatly shifts our attitudes. Davidson was trying to provide information on exactly *how* this happens. He not only discovered a variety of ways that meditation affects brain chemistry, he also found that by focusing on different imagery while in meditation your brain changes in different ways. That we can change how our brains operate simply by imagining it was groundbreaking. Science had a handle on the neural manipulation possible through physical rigor; here was proof the imagination offers similar benefits. Davidson's work has spawned numerous similar studies.

Consider compassion, a major aspect of Buddhist practice: the ability to not only empathize with another human, but to consciously choose to help them. Compassion means 'co-suffering.' You are able to understand, ideally without judgment, what another person is going through. Instead of chastising you offer a shoulder. This heart-opening practice of the Buddhist and yogi is not designed to yield karmic rewards. It is done because we're all human, we all suffer, and helping out is better than ignoring or dwelling in the details.

While meditating on compassion, Davidson's scans revealed significant activity in the insula, a region near the brain's frontal portion that plays a key role in bodily representations of emotion. This area is also activated in empathy research. Activity also increased in the temporal parietal juncture, particularly the right hemisphere. Studies have implicated this area as important in processing empathy, especially in perceiving the mental and emotional state of others.

Compassion meditation—envisioning the word and imagining yourself practicing it—strengthens the parts of your brain necessary for performing compassionate acts. Actually practicing them also strengthens those regions. You close the distance between what you choose to think and how you act. Self-study becomes an introverted and extroverted practice. You think it; you become it. Neural ties become stronger. Soon you engage every situation compassionately.

Davidson's research also found that focusing on devotion activates the visual cortex. As we discussed earlier, envisioning a physical act turns on the same neural regions as if we're actually partaking in that action. This quality is shared with music, as different styles activate our brain as if we're actually experiencing the emotion the song is invoking. Film composers, for example, are paid to create drama and anticipation with their vast repertoire of instruments and comprehension of scales and notes. You can accomplish the same emotional shifts, working through depression, anger, and uncertainty, by meditating on something you have devoted yourself to. This has long been the role of a statue or *yantra* in the yoga practice.

This is important knowledge when contemplating the self. Think of all the times you've heard, or have said, 'That's just how I'm wired!' Such thinking ranges from addictions and vices to an inability to cool off after being agitated or come down from an anxiety attack. When we habituate ourselves to respond to stimuli in a certain manner, we then think that pattern defines who we are. Our national media capitalizes on this cognitive trend by polarizing people as if being a staunch conservative or romantic liberal represents the totality of the person under investigation. Buying into the story of the one-sided self is a certain path to depression and anxiety. Meditation is a prescription that alleviates these symptoms.

First and foremost: you must sit. At the very least, question how your actions are affecting others. There are many examples of bad habits destroying habitats and communities far removed from us. The Great Pacific Vortex is an oceanic region between Hawaii and California filled with non-biodegradable plastic—up to 750,000 bits per square kilometer. Marine food webs are being decimated as sunlight no longer reaches the algae below the surface of the water, a spiral impacting the smallest to largest predators. Every time we choose a plastic bottle instead of refilling our glass we contribute to this disaster. The hard part is in understanding how seemingly small actions accumulate in major ecological crises. But they do.

Yet Americans don't necessarily have to wrap their heads around climate change as we are one of the countries that will escape most of its fury. The worst hit? India, the Pacific Islands, countries in north and eastern Africa, such as Egypt, Ethiopia, Kenya and Mozambique, as well as Suriname in South America. Nations already rural and poor are going to suffer further while America is one of the least vulnerable on the planet. If we can't see it, it must not exist. This has long been part of our social identity. In a connected world, however, we have the potential for great change, if we are willing to contemplate how we treat resources.

New York City yoga teacher Leslie Kaminoff once expressed the triad of *tapas* / *svādhyāya* / *ishvarapranidhāna* like this: *tapas* is knowing what you can change; sv*ādhyāya* is knowing what you cannot change; *ishvarapranidhāna* is understanding the difference between the two. While I've investigated sv*ādhyāya* as an inner means of recognizing what can be changed, the process would actually be accomplished through *tapas*. The two go hand-in-hand: knowledge and action. Knowing the difference between them is an important skill. And it is to that we now turn.

8 ISHVARAPRANIDHANA : A STROKE OF INSIGHT

JILL BOLTE TAYLOR wanted to understand why she can connect
her dreams with reality, and even make her dreams come true, a skill
her schizophrenic brother did not possess. She decided to study
severe mental disorders through postmortem investigation. The
neuroanatomist has since become one of the most recognized public
speakers in her field, though it took a tragedy to get her there.

On December 10, 1996, a blood vessel exploded in the left
half of Taylor's brain. She woke up to an intense pain behind her left
eye. It gripped her, then released. She attempted her morning routine
with cardiovascular exercise, until she noticed that her hands looked
like ancient claws. Suddenly her body no longer seemed like her own.
She became a witness to her own experience.

Her headache intensified. As Taylor left the exercise machine,
the fluidity of her pace weakened. Standing in her bathroom she
listened to a dialogue inside of her body: these muscles contract,
those relax. Propping herself up against a wall, her brain chatter went
silent. She was first shocked then captivated by the expansive void
inside her head.

Totally immersed in this new world of consciousness, all
boundaries dissolved. Taylor was at one with all of the energy in the
universe. She felt captivated by the molecules and atoms swirling
inside of her bathroom, in awe at the lack of brain chatter. Stress

dissipated. Peacefulness pervaded. She felt euphoric.

Then her brain's other hemisphere kicked back into gear. Her right arm went paralyzed. She realized she was having a stroke.

The oddest thought followed: she thought it was so cool that a brain scientist got the chance to study her favorite organ from the inside out.

Taylor made her way to her desk to call work. Since she couldn't remember her phone number, she pulled out a three-inch stack of business cards. Words and numbers disappeared; everything was comprised of pixels. Forty-five minutes later she was one inch down.

Since her understanding of what numbers represent was obliterated, she waited for a wave of clarity to position the phone next to the stack of cards, attempting to match the shape of the squiggles on the card to a corresponding squiggle on the keypad. Eventually she got through to a colleague. Help arrived. Despite a blood cot the size of a golf ball pressing against her brain's language center, she recovered fully.

In one of the most popular TED talks ever, 'Stroke of Insight,' Taylor discusses the differences between the brain's right and left hemispheres. This clean-cut division of labor—the right creative, the left logical—is debated by neuroscientists who recognize the interconnectivity of neural functions. The myth developed in the 1860's when it was noticed that damage to the left hemisphere radically alters language and motor control, while similar damage to the right does not. This split has made for a convenient meme, even if the truth is more nuanced. Regardless, Taylor's stroke of insight was to not rely on the intellectual academic forming the basis of her identity, and instead strive for creativity and beauty. Her realization was quite profound and beautiful.

It took one of the most daunting brain disorders for Taylor to arrive at this plateau, which she dubbed her nirvana. Trauma often serves as a gateway for life changes. Upon recovery she became devoted to this poetic lifestyle.

ISHVARAPRANIDHANA MEANS 'devotion to the Lord.' The *Yoga Bhāshya* describes it as a renunciation of all fruits of action, instead offering everything to one's conception of the divine. Interestingly, the same book claims this special kind of love (*bhakti*) causes the Lord to favor the yogi.

Etymologically it implies surrender, similar to the larger context of the word Islam. It is, as mentioned above, the third in Leslie Kaminoff's triad: knowing the difference between what you can and cannot change. Treated this way *ishvarapranidhāna* is rather challenging, as it requires taking complete responsibility for your actions, as well as controlling your response to situations beyond your control.

What are we surrendering to, however? Is it really, like Taylor suggests, an expansive world of limitless potential, or rather an altering of brain chemistry to better understand the nature of the universe? Religion, like spirituality, thrives in the realm of values. Both fall victim to overactive imaginations when metaphysics gets mixed in. While I'm a fan of the mythological rehashings of old tales—I always get choked up when Luke Skywalker stares into the horizon of Tatooine's two suns, and feel chills when the hobbits approach Sauron—I'm aware that these are works of fantasy.

Contemplating divine origins of brain matter creates a dilemma: it often stops us from doubting. While the word 'doubt' is often associated with negative consequences, from a neural perspective it's quite healthy. In Zen Buddhist practice, meditating on uncertainty helps one cultivate doubt, leading to perplexity and the crucial state of not knowing. Doubt *is* the goal, not a hindrance; it's the closest to seeing reality as it really is.

This particular strand of doubt has special meaning. According to Buddhist scholar Stephen Batchelor, "doubt dissolves into a realization that clarifies one's true 'not-knowing' nature." Batchelor believes not knowing is critical in any spiritual practice. As he writes, "To say 'I don't know' is not an admission of weakness or ignorance, but an act of truthfulness: an honest acceptance of the limits of the human condition when faced with 'the great matter of birth and death'... The willingness to embrace the fundamental bewilderment of a finite, fallible creature as the basis for leading a life that no longer clings to the superficial consolations of certainty."

Certainty among religious followers potentially leads to disaster. We don't often associate doubt—an actual process in our brains—as a form of spiritual progress. Yet doubt and disbelief have fueled some of humanity's greatest intellectual as well as ethical discoveries. Doubting is one of the most unacknowledged vehicles for innovations in politics, science and religion. If we were to historically trace doubt, we'd uncover a number of the most brilliant minds the world has ever known.

Philosophers, heretics, scientists, poets, and nearly every founder of the world's religions doubted the previous religious and social order: Socrates, Galileo, Darwin, Confucius, Schopenhauer, Karl Marx, Frederick Douglass, Emily Dickinson, St. Augustine, Stephen Hawking and George Carlin. Doubt occurs while chasing truth and exhibits profound integrity. For example, Lucretia Mott, Elizabeth Cady Stanton, and Susan B. Anthony were leaders of American feminist movements, which doubted male supremacy; all three championed the abolitionist movement that doubted the morality of slavery as well. They contemplated the theory of slavery's divine origins and rejected it, for the betterment of a nation.

Doubt involves questioning prevailing myths embedded in society as well as personal doubts (and assurances). Our brain is a fertile ground for cultivating the many beliefs it also needs to question, an intriguing conundrum: it is the instrument that thinks while thinking about itself. Doubt is a natural component of cognition. Buddhism likewise observes the transient nature of existence. Once one is too assured of a fixed belief, it is likely to change right in front of their eyes—hence the saying, 'change is the only constant.'

Interestingly, our brain believes everything first presented to it. Then it must decide whether or not it's true. There's an incredible array of neural processes taking place in order for us to doubt. In just the last few years we began to understand what a brain must do to determine whether something is true or false.

Antonio Damasio calls the process of doubting 'false tagging.' This recent theory has created an expanding field of research in neuroscience. The area of the brain we use to doubt or false tag has been pinpointed in the prefrontal cortex—specifically the ventromedial prefrontal cortex (vmPFC). This is the region where we make decisions and respond to emotions and feelings.

Research conducted at the University Of Iowa determined that the initial step of understanding something is inseparable from believing it; only a secondary psychological act can produce disbelief or doubt. This model asserts that belief occurs in two stages: mental representation and assessment. A mental representation of an idea, initially regarded as true, must be tagged to indicate false value. The prefrontal cortex is necessary for the false tag, which is comprised of affective states that are emotional in nature.

We first feel an idea emotionally. We then need a healthy prefrontal cortex to judge its validity. In one study patients with damage to the vmPFC were roughly twice as likely to believe an ad even when shown disclaimer information pointing out its falsity. They were also more likely to buy the item, regardless of whether misleading information had been corrected.

In another study research showed damage to this specific region promotes religious fundamentalism. Study participants—similar across groups in age, gender and religious affiliation—filled out a survey measuring how extreme their religious beliefs were. Another survey gauged the extent to which their personalities could be described as authoritarian, while a third questionnaire asked whether patients' beliefs in four specific Christian doctrines had changed since their injury. As investigators expected, participants who had experienced damage to their vmPFC showed significantly higher levels of fundamentalist beliefs than those in two control groups. They also reported greater increases in religious belief since their injury, as well as higher levels of authoritarianism.

Is religious belief merely the product of a malfunctioning doubt mechanism in the prefrontal cortex? That's doubtful. It isn't as simple as one neural region, though the study implies that extreme religious beliefs are easier to entertain if a person has a decreased ability to doubt these beliefs. It also shows the importance of questioning *any* belief.

In our quest for meaning we ask whether the universe has a hidden agenda, whether someone cares about our stories, who we are and where we're going. Evidence suggests we are the only ones who care. We have to ask ourselves if it's the cosmic questions or the seemingly simpler ones that are relevant. Are we really a creator's special creature, justified in destroying entire ecosystems, ravaging foreign lands, and killing tens of billions of animals every year because a special entity gave us permission? Oftentimes our divine inheritance sounds more like a bank robbery.

Religion has done positive things for people. Unfortunately cynicism and nihilism are sometimes the result of people being fed up with faith. I'm not arguing for that kind of rejection. There are states of mind and ways of being that I gladly affix the term spiritual to. I simply do not believe that being a moral and just person requires supernatural influence. That said, if someone's belief system helps him or her be better, wonderful.

Two problems often arise from this, however. First, if an individual preaches one thing but acts in a completely opposite matter, he is ripe for a neuroses and crisis of character. And two, it allows people to escape confrontational emotions and assign divine purpose to it, such as the escalating skirmishes in Israel. When Israelis and Palestinians no longer see one another as human beings, it's easy to go to battle. And while human psychology might be at the origins of such battles—we'll discuss the concept of disgust in the next chapter—this war, among many others, is waged under the banner of religion: one tribe not doubting its divine inheritance.

Most people I know reject this form of religion. Yet we

cannot turn a blind eye to the fact that for many people it really is a function of their faith. Having studied religious and ethnic conflicts for decades, I began wondering not what people believe, but *why* we believe in the first place. And that question is being answered.

AUTOBIOGRAPHY OF A YOGI remains an influential book in yoga circles. Numerous teacher trainings use it in their curriculum. Its author, Paramahansa Yogananda, founded the Self Realization Fellowship in 1920, opening doors at the Los Angeles location five years later. It is estimated that he introduced millions of westerners to meditation and kriya yoga through this famous book, first published in 1946.

One scene in the predominantly anecdotal work stands out: Yogananda is walking with his teacher who, to show the power of the soul over the body, reportedly leaves his skin and assumes the flesh of a dead man. It reminds one of Krishna discussing the godhead taking off and putting on bodies as humans do with clothes in the *Bhagavad Gītā*. Yogananda was not the first or last to make such a claim. The idea of an animated spirit residing inside of this fleshly container is very old indeed.

The soul is a seductive notion. Many believe the 'I' inside the 'me' is an ethereal element, not confined by laws of physiology or biology. Instead the murky term energy is employed to describe the perceived limitless bounds of imagination we use when we conjure past lives, have out-of-body experiences and feel tiny prickles of light. Coincidences are never what they seem, for they must be destined messages from a wise and knowledgeable beyond conducting the orchestrations of the universe from somewhere far away, yet always near. This soul is our true home, the world of flesh and politics and mortgages and disease all part of the cosmic play confusing us to our true nature.

While science is often perceived as the antithesis, and therefore the enemy, of such thinking, there is no consensus of what scientists believe. They are dualists as often as atheists. Some believe an ineffable source influences and directs brain functions, while others view consciousness purely as a function of chemistry. There is no agreed upon view. Yet to not investigate how our brain works is lazy. Saying that since we don't know something then we should assign it to an unknown divinity lacks integrity, leading to a shedding of personal responsibility. If we think something is meant to be, we can write it off as a cosmic sign instead of following through with whatever we intended to accomplish. It is the easy way out.

A disembodied soul neatly fills in gaps in our thinking. We despise incomplete stories. Remember, our brains evolved to notice patterns in nature. If we cannot recognize one clearly, we'll invent it. Personal satisfaction trumps mystery. Let's return to the doctor's office. You immediately want to know what's wrong. Waiting time between tests is torturous; your brain creates all sorts of explanations. If your doctor cannot explain the illness, or if he gives you a diagnosis you didn't want to hear, you might seek out a second opinion. And third. And so on.

This kind of rigor is sometimes necessary when dealing with our bodies, especially given how commonly misdiagnoses occur. The quest for the soul is fundamentally different. Knowledge of a spirit 'out there' satisfies a certain emotional intelligence, comforts one into thinking something greater is on their team. We feel wanted; death no longer frightens us. If reincarnation is a fact, why worry about little things? We'll come back, anyway. If something watching over us is concerned with our greatest good, why fret over mundane trifles? We're loved, somewhere, even if not here, now. Such a balm is addictive.

But is this habit of disassociating an imaginary soul from the biological mechanisms nature has endowed us with part of our genetic inheritance? Turns out that might be the case. As Paul Bloom points out, babies have two inherent systems that have been adapted to promote the belief that such a soul lives inside of us.

For quite some time the blank slate theory dominated: we are born into this world with a clean canvas. All of our vices, brilliance, passions, and bigotry are learned through society, parents and teachers. Now we know better than that. Babies, Bloom's area of expertise, are born with the notion that there is a 'me' occupying the body it is inside. This is partly due to our comprehension of the social world, which evolves at a different pace than our understanding of the physical world.

When we gaze at babies and wonder what they 'know,' it turns out quite more than we believed. If you show a six-month-old an object on a table, and then pull the table away and the object is suspended in the air (via a hidden string), the baby is surprised. He understands gravity. Babies can also do simple math, understand pleasure and disgust, and display preferences for people they perceive as kind while shying away from those they have observed doing harm to others. Bloom likens the difference between a baby's social and physical world as two separate computers running in the baby's brain. Their social world emerges after the world of objects and flesh. (Autism is an extreme example of the development of the physical world without social adaptation.) This distance between two different worlds might explain why we separate an invisible entity from the all-too-real existence of bones and blood. The ghost in the machine is a feature, not an anomaly.

What kind of existence this soul embodies and how it moves about in the afterlife is the product of cultures. This is the realm of mythologies: an ability to travel to future times, dismembered gods being put back together, goddesses living in the underworld during winter, the three-tiered universe of shamans, spiritual leaders bouncing from existence to existence in mountaintop kingdoms. In general children believe in this disembodied person phenomena more than adults, but judging by international poll results, the majority of humans seek some sort of inner peace through such an idea. They simply cannot perceive existence any other way. Previous and future lives appeal to our primitive emotions, the thrust for survival and procreation. If in this physical world we can leave a genetic legacy behind, why wouldn't we leave a spiritual identity in our wake as well?

This leads to our body's second system of supernatural exploitation: personification. We see humanity in everything. Clouds display human faces. Children talk to dolls and stuffed animals, naming them as they would a pet. We personify all of existence to serve our needs and give us purpose.

Before Darwin every culture had some sense of intentional design. Polytheistic gods were always destroying and recreating and saving villages and worlds. Then the monotheistic God came along and consistently chose one side over the other—whatever side was writing Him into existence. Epic disasters and tragedies were designed to teach people a lesson. Slowly animal gods assumed human form, at first mutant half-bulls, half-humans and so forth. The role of divinity went from the natural world around us to humans controlling that world through divine intervention. Virgin and animal sacrifices transformed into the interior world of prayer and intention. The ways we communicated with an ethereal energy changed, but the fact that we talk to an intervening agent did not. And whatever face or faceless form that agent assumed, he was there for a human purpose.

Darwin threw a wrench into all that. Natural selection no longer needed a divine overseer tinkering at the controls. His theories influenced our understanding of science greatly, but as Bloom points out, the idea makes no *intuitive sense*—and as Jonathan Haidt argues, we are driven by intuition before reason. If life is all about making sure human beings get what they want, an absentee creator demolishes the very foundation of that desire.

From the viewpoint of children, everything has a reason for existing. As Bloom writes, "When asked to explain why a bunch of rocks are pointy, adults prefer a physical explanation, while children choose a functional one, such as 'so that animals could scratch on them when they get itchy.' And when asked about the origins of animals and people, children tend to prefer explanations that involve an intentional creator, even if the adults raising them do not.

Creationism—and belief in God—is bred in the bone."

The last two centuries of scientific inquiry has overturned much of our understanding of how the world works. Yet our belief in disembodiment persists. While some understand evolutionary biology and neuroscience, they don't *feel* that's how the world works, and so they reject the possibility that their instinct might be wrong. In fact, that's one of the most common phrases I've heard in my twenty-one years of practicing yoga: you have to *feel* instead of *think*. The emotional body is more knowledgeable than the intellectual mind. There must be some cosmic energy influencing our daily lives and destiny, right?

Writer and political activist Barbara Ehrenreich decided to test this hypothesis. She looked into conflated claims that the law of attraction was scientifically provable. First she investigated if gravity is responsible for binding invisible thoughts with visible reality, in which she concluded, "One, thoughts are not objects with mass; they are patterns of neuronal firing within the brain. Two, if they were exerting some sort of gravitational force on material objects around them, it would be difficult to take off one's hat." This would also be the case with souls carrying a lifetime of memories from body to body.

Next she tackled the notion that thoughts are positive or negative vibrations. Mantra singers sometimes make this claim. Sanskrit syllables are supposedly heavenly revelations connecting us with a universal force, while low energy statements like gossip and curse words prohibit us from divine association. Thoughts, however, are not vibrations either. She compares them with sound waves, which *are* vibrations characterized by amplitude and frequency. There is no positive or negative correlation to actual vibrations.

Magnetism is one popular catchphrase from this ideological camp. Ehrenreich concedes that thoughts do indeed produce electrical activity and generate a magnetic field—an extremely weak field, however. If our brains could produce a field strong enough to leave our skulls, magnets would fly off the refrigerator every time we walked by. The earth's magnetic field, which is where these thoughts (or souls) would have to have influence, is 10,000,000,000 times more powerful than that of our brain.

Critical thinking and talk of the soul are often set at odds. When I've mentioned research like the above, I've been criticized for being negative, not open-minded enough to see the possibilities of transmigration and divine intervention. My answer is always the same: show me proof and I'll change my narrative. It's changed frequently over the years. I too bought into reincarnation and the buddy upstairs until I began investigating how our brains operate. Another key for me was studying history. I know plenty of yogis who read spiritual texts but never open history books. You cannot understand philosophical ideas without diving into the social, political, and economic conditions that influenced the tribes and nations that produced them. Repeating what you want to be true simply because you desire life to be that way does not reflect the world we actually live in.

This is not to say that any of the qualities discussed above are not healthy. Being positive, empathetic, and caring is important. Maintaining an optimistic outlook helps us deal with emotionally challenging times, as well as offering compassion to those in need of it. Recall my doctor friend informing me of the importance of attitude when dealing with cancer. I took time out every day during the process of recovery, post-surgery and through chemotherapy, to remember everything I'm grateful for. Such an attitude has been shown to have remarkable benefits.

Dr. Robert Emmons at the University of California, Davis spent eight years intensively studying gratitude. His research found having an attitude of gratitude improves emotional and physical health, as well as strengthens relationships and communities. One of the greatest challenges is overcoming the victim mentality so prominent in our species, as well as moving beyond a sense of entitlement or ownership. Implementing daily thankfulness empowers us. It is much more beneficial than believing that we're owed something, or that some illusive energy is out to get us. Both of those mindsets imply that an energetic force is responsible for the direction of our lives, which is another way of shirking responsibility for our actions. Gratitude enables us to take charge of how we exist in this world without the seesaw of pride and defeat.

One of Emmons's studies found that people who kept a gratitude journal exercise more frequently, report fewer physical symptoms of pain, and are more optimistic about the upcoming week, compared to those who kept neutral journals. He also discovered those keeping gratitude lists made greater strides in progressing toward personal goals over a two-month period.

In another study with young adults practicing daily gratitude exercises, those who partook reported higher levels of alertness, enthusiasm, determination, attentiveness, and energy compared to the control group, who were either told to focus on downward social comparisons or that they were better off than others.

Expressing gratitude appears to have strong ties with overall life satisfaction. After a series of gratitude visits, in which people wrote a letter and then delivered it to someone who had helped them substantially at some point in their lives, their happiness scores rose by 10% and depression scores dropped significantly. Gratitude appears to be uniquely important for both psychological wellbeing and in social relationships.

Which is the thrust of *ishvarapranidhāna*. We can be devoted without needing to be devoted *to* something. There is no end to what we can aim our allegiance at: using less resources, being more considerate of others, eating better, exercising, smiling more. As mentioned in the Introduction, yoga is a discipline that must be regularly practiced if it's going to be effective. If we devote our lives to yoga, we are really training our brains to pursue the moral codes Patanjali set down to page all those years ago. Actively changing what we can is an important component; relieving ourselves of anxiety over what we cannot is the other half. As for the difference between? We all hope our practice will reveal what is true, the pursuit of which we now turn.

9 SATYA : THE ETERNAL QUEST

ODDLY, RAILROADS PLAY an important role in moral tales. You might have heard this one: You're standing next to a railroad switch as a speeding train barrels toward five people trapped on the tracks. If you pull the lever, you'll force the train to switch tracks; on the second a lone person is stranded. You either let the train run its course and kill five people, or you intervene and only one person dies.

Most people pull the lever. From a genetic standpoint, saving five lives is better for our species than one. Yet you probably don't think of it from that perspective. Most likely you consider a different cost-benefit analysis: five families versus one, five husbands or wives, children and so on. Since no one is related to you there is no specific emotional draw. It's merely numbers, irrespective of how you later justify the decision.

There is a second scenario with the same outcome. Only this time you're standing on a bridge overlooking the tracks. Once again five people (who probably should have learned their lesson) are stranded. Now a large man is standing next to you. You can push him off the bridge and save five lives. (Suicide is not an option since you are not big enough to stop the train.) Do you make the same decision?

Of course not.

Hypotheticals do not necessarily reflect reality. The odds of ever being in either situation are miniscule, much less both. Nothing could ever replace actually being in a position that requires split-second decision-making. Joseph Campbell writes about a man who risked his own life saving another person. At that moment, the lifesaver said, no other option seemed possible. He *had* to act. Campbell deposited this tale in the realm of the mythological, where time seems to slow to an excruciating rate and we move with *Matrix*-like precision. Intuition trumps reason.

We may claim that we would risk our life to save a stranger, yet in the moment, another reality might unfold. A recent circus video went viral in which two lions began attacking their captors inside of the cage. While no one ended up hurt (save the lions, who were prodded with sharp sticks and shot with fire hoses), most intriguing was the crowd. As soon as everyone realized the lions were not playing by the rules, they quickly filed out of their seats—not toward the ring, mind you. Even though the fifteen-foot high cage separated cat from man, they weren't taking chances.

Recall the meme of our brain's halves divided into the boring, colorless logical side and the psychedelic creative way more interesting brother. While misleading, it does imply an inherent rift inside of us. We like to think of ourselves as moral beings. Yet we fool ourselves time and again. Our better angels would never survive without our demons.

SATYA MEANS 'TRUTH.' This *yama* is related to *ahimsa*; lying causes harm. The yoga texts tend to focus on speaking truthfully. For example, the *Garuda Purāna* deems *satya* 'speech that is beneficial to beings.' There is also a sense of portraying truth in action and thought as well. Truth does, at times, get mixed in with mysticism: the *Yoga Sutras* declares that practicing truth empowers the yogi with paranormal powers (*siddhis*), while the *Yoga Bhāsya* states that being truthful will make everything you say come true—an ancient version of *The Secret*, I suppose.

There are two layers in understanding the concept of truth. The first concerns lying. Seems pretty clear-cut. If you know you are telling a falsehood, don't do it, right? For example, say you've been cheating on your partner. They confront you about this. Is it better to reveal your infidelity in hopes of salvaging the relationship or live with the guilt of knowing that you've lied? Will telling the truth help end what was not going well anyway? Or is deception worthwhile, as you figure you can get away with it through sweet words and comfort sex? Do you realize this might be your last chance: you don't reveal the affair, though you end it to avoid further potential harm?

From the perspective of *satya*, you tell the truth. Not only do you reveal the reality of your sexual misgivings (assuming you and your partner were both on board for monogamy), but you also explore the feelings associated with your decision for straying. You put everything on the table and see what the next step is. This is certainly the quickest route to healing. Everyone is on the same page. There will be pain, but there will no longer be deceit.

Lying also stunts our imagination. We can no longer speak freely. If we are honest with people, we never have to backtrack to remember what story we're telling. We speak our mind without worry. When we lie, however, we have to constantly recall who we told what. Our storytelling ability is damaged by the persistent necessity of juggling numerous tales in our mind at once, keeping us on perpetual guard. Many lies are exposed due to a misstep in chronology, as you no longer remember who did what when.

The path of deceit also harms friendships. Research has shown that liars trust those who believe their lies less than they otherwise would. If they fell for it, the logic goes, they are not worth trusting. The lack of trust you have in yourself is transferred outwardly. Everything and everyone, over time, is viewed through this clouded lens. The falsities you've created become a full-time occupation.

Yet lying is not always so explicit. Say you have a friend who is a struggling yoga instructor. She's been teaching for five years but nothing seems to go her way. She's unable to bring in a sustainable number of students and continually loses classes. Online reviews are not glowing. Perhaps she's too tough, or too much of a pushover, or doesn't project her voice enough. Maybe people can't stand her music selection. There are many variables. Do you encourage her to keep trying regardless of the results? Implore her to continue to follow her passion, even if her presentation is obviously flawed?

Neuroscientist and author Sam Harris argues that this sort of false encouragement "is a kind of theft: it steals time, energy, and motivation a person could put toward some other purpose." Yoga instruction in a group setting is, among other things, a performance. The lighting, sound, tone and timbre of your voice, and overall flow of your class are parts comprising the entire experience. Early, albeit brief, training in theater during college taught me how to project my voice properly, a skill I later applied when I began teaching. Would you suggest a public speaking class to your friend if that was her problem, or instead say ignore the critics and plow ahead?

Harris believes that deceiving a friend is a form of lying. "When we presume to lie for the benefit of others, we have decided that *we* are the best judges of how much they should understand about their own lives... What attitude could be more disrespectful of those we care about?"

Only we know our friends, and each friend is different. I worked for many years as a music critic. Criticism is important: it serves as a mirror for artists and creators to gauge their work. Not all criticism is warranted, and much of it, especially in the age of blog comments, should be ignored. I don't know how many times people have commented on an article of mine without actually reading it. Others use that section to sound off with their own emotional or mental issues regardless of whether it has anything to do with the content. Still others have operated in the same role I attempt when writing about music: as a reflection that serves to strengthen the overall argument, or as a call to change course due to conflicting evidence. This form of debate is healthy, and ideally should be applied when dealing with friends who might need a helping hand…or words. If they are disgusted by helpful criticism, then you have to question the strength of your friendship in the first place.

This outward lying is an important facet of *satya*. We will explore another more insidious form during the rest of this chapter. Before we get there, let us first visit an important word just invoked to dig a little deeper into our humanity.

AS PAUL BLOOM WRITES, disgust has long played an important role in our species. The emotion helps us navigate the treacherous terrain of poisonous and spoiled foods. The upturned nose when smelling rotten fruit and inquisitive eyebrow expressing uncertainty in regards to the mushroom beneath your feet helps us avoid ingesting toxic substances.

Disgust was not only in response to food. It also applied to pathogens and bacteria. The smell of an unclean person disgusts us, Bloom writes, because it reveals disease. In biological terms, avoiding that which could kill us makes sense, whether via food poisoning or catching whatever that unkempt villager has. Over time we made a cognitive leap to apply this survival mechanism to human sexuality.

Outside of hygienic concerns, having sex with animals should not disgust us, he explains, at least if done in private (leaving aside concern for the animal's welfare). Yet it does. The same goes for incest. Genetically incest is unhealthy, but that's not why we cringe when thinking about sleeping with a sibling—unless, of course, you're in *Game of Thrones* and have kings to produce. Sex with siblings and animals makes us feel icky. We don't consider another person engaging in such sexual acts as much as we mentally put ourselves in the position of doing so. Mirror neurons meet imagination.

Most species of animals do not crossbreed. We are (hopefully) attracted to other human beings. As for incest, this is predominantly through moral codes taught to us. It was not always considered weird, especially if you lived your entire life in a village of 150 people or less, as our ancestors did for most of human history.

Much of what we consider cringe worthy is due to social conditioning.

Disgust plays a more important role in perceived deviance, however. The most prominent civil right of our era is marriage equality. Homosexuality is arguably as old as we are. While the more devout might claim it has always been sinful, many societies have if not embraced it at least not admonished it the way we have over the last century. We protest priests having sex with teenage boys, but this was once common practice. The word 'pederasty' comes from the Greek *paiderastia* and means 'love of boys.' In Athens in the sixth century BCE this form of sex was enjoyed, not considered an abomination to be avoided.

America celebrates plenty of perversions while shunning the natural love between two people, regardless of sexual preference. As Bloom notes, homosexual activity should not disgust us. If anything, only women should be upset by two men having sex, as it pulls them out of the gene pool. The same applies to men and lesbians, but given our many sexual double standards, this is rarely the case.

A double standard was recently witnessed in the Supreme Court decision on *Burwell v. Hobby Lobby*, in which the justices voted to allow companies to patrol what forms of birth control its employees were purchasing, denying them the rights to buy four types that supposedly offended the owner's religious beliefs. From the outset the case was flawed. The argument hinged on the fact that those four were abortifacients, an entirely false claim. The fact this whole ordeal had nothing to do with religion became clear a day after the case was decided when investigative reporting revealed that Hobby Lobby invested more than $73 million in companies producing the very birth control products it was denying its employees access to.

That same day Michael Wear, who directed President Obama's faith outreach campaign in 2012, requested that companies be exempt from partaking in the president's planned legislation banning discrimination against the LGBT community. Obama's new initiative states that if companies receive federal contracts they cannot use sexual preference as grounds for not hiring someone. Wear's justification is religious.

The sexual preference argument is presented as a moral one. Opponents of gay marriage, for example, claim that their religion's ethical guidelines prohibit this sort of behavior. Yet this does not make sense. As Blooms writes, "The mystery for moral psychologists isn't why we would engage in certain types of sex while avoiding other types; it's why we should be so concerned with the sex that other people are having."

Anti-gay marriage advocates rely on invoking disgust to present their platform. If homosexuality is perceived as sinful and savage, followers will dehumanize anyone believing otherwise. The same holds true with abortion and, incredibly, birth control. In research Bloom conducted with colleagues, he found aversion to topics like abortion and gay marriage were more often associated with people who express a range of politically conservative ideas. Yet another study showed having strong disgust sensitivity in general equates to expressing revulsion to homosexuality and other sex-related activities even among liberal thinkers. Like conspiracy theorists buying into numerous conspiracies once their brain is open to one, easily disgusted humans begin to feel revulsion in regards to other topics. What it essentially comes down to is *purity*.

Consider body fluids. Most invoke disgust. Walk by a puddle of urine. Watch snot fly from someone's nose. Vomit. (Interestingly tears are excluded.) This is why, Bloom believes, religions have produced a variety of cleansing techniques to make their followers pure. Christian baptism and ritual Islamic washing (*wudu*) are two examples. Joseph Campbell believes this to be a longstanding feature of cultures, beginning with infants presenting their feces as gifts. Parents quickly attempt to dissuade this act. Yet this psychological phenomenon of cleanliness exists at the foundation of numerous mythological motifs. Hell is a place of filth, heaven the Disneyworld of the cosmos.

Today we don't need ritual paints when Photoshop magically clears up any blemishes when presenting our selfies to the world. Yet we apply 'clean' and 'dirty' to a range of practices, not just our bodies. Take language. One study showed that people expressing malicious lies over the phone chose mouthwash as a parting gift; another group, which had to lie over email, chose hand sanitizer.

While innate, disgust is a learned behavior within cultural parameters. The smell of durian, for example, makes me want to run far away, while one of my best friends can't wait to shove it down his throat. Exposure breeds tolerance. Surround yourself with a community of others who think abortion is an offense, or that homosexual activity is sacrilegious, and your disgust turns to revulsion. The 'others' are no longer even human in your eyes. Their rights become inconsequential. When contemplating social policy this is tragic. What this sort of thinking leads to—insert ethnic cleansing here—is atrocious.

Americans like to think themselves above such potential catastrophes. Given that national polls are in favor of same-sex marriages and most citizens support women's rights, I doubt internment camps will be set up for homosexuals. Other countries, of course, are not so fortunate. Even still, in a time when anyone can have a blog and most lunatics do, the separation between 'them' and 'us' handicaps us as a nation. Whenever there is an opportunity to turn a group of people with opposing views into the 'other,' philosophical and moral rifts split wide apart.

Which is why talk of this being about religious freedom is nonsense. Proponents of anti-LGBT and –birth control measures are using faith to hide behind their mask of bias—a learned bias, not a divine mandate. Their religious road to freedom leads to its own prison, one that over time, if fed and nurtured, runs into similar nationalistic cleansing efforts any sane man or woman is disgusted by when studying history. Ironically, religionists believe homosexuality is learned and can therefore be unlearned. In fact, only two states in the union—my home state of New Jersey and my current residence,

California—have banned reparative therapy for minors. That is, curing the gay away. It's still legal in the other forty-eight.

Sexual preference has long been shown to be innate. What we learn are biases, such as those against homosexuality. *That* actually can be unlearned. We need to use all of our sciences to understand how we create morals. As we've seen, disgust is one powerful catalyst for the ethical mind.

The question we now need to face is a hard one. Yet I don't think it should remain unasked. In fact, Sam Harris did a wonderful job of addressing this issue in *The Moral Landscape*. Can we scientifically address our moral dilemmas?

TO UNDERSTAND OURSELVES consider genetic divergence, a process in which species split apart. This usually occurs after one subpopulation has lived in isolation for many generations in an entirely different environment. As science writer Virginia Morell writes, "Evolution is not linear. It is divergent—which means that we all sit on the limbs of a bushy tree, each species as evolved as the next, the anatomical differences largely a result of ecology and behavior."

Divergence often takes place over the length of thousands and tens of thousands of years. No single lifespan could account for the development of a brain as complex and nuanced as ours. You've probably heard the saying that our time here on earth is as brief as the blink of an eye. While there's a lot of truth in this, we don't often feel it to be the case.

Thus the emergence of creation mythology. Every recorded culture in history has had one. Maoris believe a bird dropped an egg into the primeval sea and out popped a man and woman, their two children, a pig, a dog, and, obviously, a canoe—how else would they have navigated the oceanic terrain? New Zealand is a world removed from Siberia, however, where ancient Kamchatkans thought God got bored in heaven and paid earth a visit. Apparently the planet was very smooth, so when the big guy stepped on the land with his snowshoes valleys formed around mountains.

It would have been odd for the Maoris' conception of divinity to walk about in snowshoes considering their climate, just as a vast ocean would likely not appear in northern Russian mythology. Consider the many flood myths of India and the Middle East. Then find out what rivers these writers lived near while putting paint to rock to express their ideas of creation.

We are no different today. With a short life span on an ancient planet there is plenty of room for an imaginative play to be performed in our heads. Children do not need to be told tales of psychic witches and astral travel when they can type a few words on a screen and receive an instant answer from a distant friend. Their mythologies will be vastly different from even ours, as will their children's. Our beliefs are framed by the world we're brought up in, wildly divergent even in the same era. Imagine the different perceptions between a child brought up on the Upper East Side by millionaires and one raised in the rural Delta with no access to computers.

Religion has long been thought to be ground zero for morals. There is support for this: charity organizations are most often attached to a church, and religious congregations sometimes provide the only homeless outreach and food kitchens in town. They are usually the first to raise funds for international tragedies. These are all beautiful human acts. They just don't need religion to be accomplished. It's really the sense of community these institutions provide that matters.

As we've explored throughout this book, our brains are responsible for all of our actions and reactions, to emotions, to events, to people, likes and dislikes. We live in an age in which scientists and researchers are figuring out the neural mechanisms explaining a wide scope of biological processes. No, it's not a perfect science, and yes, we will fumble along the way. If we want to take global culture seriously, an idea expressed when yogis exclaim 'we are all one' and chant mantras of unification, we must begin on the ground floor. We have to consider a science of ethics.

Sam Harris attempted this exact task. He argued that morals have a scientific basis, and that, while still in its nascent phase, ethical guidelines striving for the greatest good for as many people as possible can be a reality. This is impossible in a climate charged with religious fervor and tribal mentality, though. We need to listen to and understand one another for this to be possible. One thousand soapboxes for every thousand people will never do.

Let's be honest: all gods were created by the human imagination. It's what our brains do. And every one of them was dreamed up to reflect the society and ecology surrounding them. No religion or spirituality has ever been static; all have changed with the times, as have the ethics associated with them. Just as same sex marriage rights are becoming ubiquitous in America today, other movements have changed societies throughout history. Our gods always change with us.

Yet still we're plagued with a brand of passivity called moral relativism: other religions have the right to practice what they want in accordance with their beliefs. While this sounds lovely on the page— in certain situations it is important—turning a blind eye in the name of faith is tragic. Arguments have been made that the genital mutilation of teenage girls in Africa should not be obstructed if done in accordance with local customs. The same holds true of women's and children's rights across the planet. There is no possible good in ruining a young woman's ability to express herself sexually. This medical atrocity is certain to scar her psychologically and physically. No benevolent god would invent such a cruel punishment. This monstrous thinking belongs to the human domain alone.

Double standards are found throughout history's religious canon. We need to turn back no further than the modern Catholic Church, an entity that prides itself on being the world's premier upholder of morals. As Harris states, "the Vatican is an organization that excommunicates women for attempting to become priests but does not excommunicate male priests for raping children. It excommunicates doctors who perform abortions to save a mother's life—even if the mother is a *nine-year-old girl raped by her stepfather and pregnant with twins*—but it did not excommunicate a single member of the Third Reich for committing genocide." The Church is not alone in such hideous contradictions: conflicting tales of liberation and oppression exist across the board.

The challenge in creating a scientific basis for morals resides in our ability to contemplate our actions and admit that we've been doing things wrong, then change how we act, if called for. As Harris writes, just because something is hard does not mean we shouldn't try to weed through the verbiage of mysticism and arrive at substantial conclusions benefiting the greatest number of people. My social media feed is bombarded by a brand of self-help lingo already hinting at this: to find the light you must walk through darkness; the hardest things are the most rewarding; being challenged lets you know you're on the right path. The individual liberties we take pride in are useless if the bulk of this planet cannot wake up peacefully in the morning.

While we're not built for imagining the suffering of the rest of the planet, that does not mean we cannot steel ourselves with empathy and compassion in our personal practice. We'll investigate how to do this in the last chapter. It involves a rewiring of neural patterns, which implies our brain maps had to be wired a certain way in the first place. As in all the other complex systems in our brain, there is no singular belief center. Harris did find that the insula plays a role in the formation of beliefs, interestingly also the region dealing with disgust. The insula also handles pain perception, empathy, humiliation and a variety of other emotions.

Evolved as a result of genetic divergence, the higher-level layers of our brain that deal with cognitive activities are the result of lower-order emotional processing; beliefs were not suddenly implanted by an external source. They are the natural result of a self-aware creature attempting to create a narrative of existence. Our brain was not built to read, for example. This skill was imagined and acquired through hundreds of thousands of years of evolution. Reading seems natural to us today, but only if we actually learn how to read. Illiterate folk would challenge the naturalness of this action.

To test how our brain creates beliefs, Harris scanned volunteers with fMRI technology as part of his doctoral research program at UCLA. He verified Spinoza's belief that "merely understanding a statement entails the tacit acceptance of its being true, while disbelief requires a subsequent process of rejection." This is similar to research cited above from the University Of Iowa and Damasio's concept of false tagging. Harris's work uncovered greater activity in the medial prefrontal cortex, a region that aids in linking factual knowledge with corresponding emotional associations. It also plays into goal-based actions and altering your behavior in response to rewards. The MPFC helps us monitor reality as well. When injuries occur in this region people have been found to lie through their teeth without realizing it. This might help explain why humans believe a lunatic screaming with conviction over a sane man speaking in a monotone, uncertain voice.

The MPFC is also responsible for self-representation. Harris thinks this is where the emotional nature of belief takes hold. If we believe something to be true, we invest ourselves in the idea. We mentally embody the hypothesis until it is woven into the fabric of our being. The MPFC, Harris writes, creates an "anatomical bridge between reasoning and value." The mental distance between rationalization and belief is obscured due to this process. The conviction of faith takes root; there will be no dismissing the validity of the belief, which has now become truth—only the truth of a brain map, not necessarily the reality the brain is attempting to understand.

What distance is there between personal perception and reality to begin with? A recent study on vaccines helps us to understand this. Over the last decade a growing anti-vaccination movement has emerged in the United States, sending school districts into a panic. A research team based at Dartmouth mailed four separate types of pro-vaccination literature to nearly 2,000 parents.

One stated that there has been no scientific evidence relating vaccines to autism, the idea that jumpstarted anti-vaccine protests; another highlighted the dangers of the diseases vaccines prevent; the third featured photos of children suffering from said diseases; the final was a story about an infant who almost died from measles. The team spent three years on the research and was startled to discover...nothing.

It didn't matter what leaflet each parent received. If they were predisposed to believing vaccines are evil, they did not change their mind, regardless of what any government agency claimed or how many photographs of sick children they saw. The neural connection—vaccines are bad—was so wired that no amount of contradictory evidence sufficed. If anything, opposing literature only fueled their resistance in what is known as the backfire effect: you say do this, I do that instead. Everyone likes to play the martyr sometimes.

It would be nice to imagine that during a time when so much information is widely available, we would self-correct. The opposite has occurred. Since anyone can have a decent looking website spouting whatever information they want to transmit, we live in an extremely polarized society. Misinformation has no actual credibility, but if it has an emotional appeal—if someone relates the information to a part of their identity—it will easily trump facts. Perhaps there has never been a truth that we all own together. Finding one would be like discovering an eternally elusive needle in the largest haystack ever pitched by mankind.

The realm of the personal blog reveals this trend. An entire literature now exists in which people take things personally or encourage others not to take things personally. We invest so much energy in our identity that anything suggesting the construction might be a façade is immediately rejected. By recognizing this we've hit upon one of the key failures of modern yoga: it is a bolstering of the ego, through selfies and self-affirmations feeding the appetite of this primeval, insatiable desire for gratification and acknowledgement. We are born deceivers, the devil resting on the shoulder opposite the angel. We are also born exhibitionists who care way more about the ego we are supposedly trying to shed through this little thing called yoga.

And it is here we find the cure next to the disease. For the techniques devised to calm that unfettered appetite are the same as they have been for thousands of years. In this we connect the ancient past with modern yoga. The concept of truth has always been a ruse; no one said self-investigation would be easy. We may never hit upon a *satya* for all of humanity. What we can learn is to be content with how we arrived at this point, using this practice as a foundation for constructive change. If this doesn't sound glamorous or sexy, that's just fine, for the heart and soul of yoga reside in accepting the present moment for what it is and moving forward from that space.

10 SANTOSHA : COMING HOME

MONDAY, APRIL 21, 2014. After finishing lunch, I noticed something strange while in the bathroom. My right testicle was swollen and hard. While I wouldn't receive verification until after a CT scan the following day, I immediately knew my life was about to change. Two hours after feeling the lump I was lying in my doctor's office, her face revealing what my instincts had intuited.

Cancer is a scary word. Granted, it's much less frightening than when I was a child, though not all cancers are created equal. While odd to write, I felt relieved that I had the most treatable form of cancer in men. Little had I known in the early eighties, when I received a series of hormone shots to fix an undescended testicle, I would most likely get cancer later in life. At the time doctors didn't know either.

The online response was tremendous. My singular blog post about the issue, written just to let a few friends know what was happening, received over 100,00 views. I lost track of email well wishes, posts of compassion and caring. The whole ordeal reminded me of the positive aspects of social media and the Internet. In times of tragedy people put aside petty differences in the hopes of sustaining life. It might be our genetic inheritance, but it is also part of who we are as social animals. As human beings. A beautiful part.

For the most part I ignored the occasional lunatic comment

as I went through the process of healing, first with surgery, then chemotherapy. Some people believe cancer is caused by the mind due to emotional suppression and felt little need to censor. I reminded myself of the anti-vaccination crowd: facts do nothing to dissuade a lack of empathy. You have to put it into perspective. They are filling in their own gaps to a story they don't understand, verifying their take by recalling it to short-term memory every time the word cancer appears. We all have patterns. Discipline involves choosing what thoughts to let in and let go of, which to strengthen and destroy.

I don't have much in this world, but what I do have was enough to help me in a time of need: good health coverage, great friends and an amazing family. Yet a lot of people have trouble reaching out for help when they need it most. While there are innumerable reasons for feeling lonely and isolated or being unable to cry out when tears are relentless, the last *niyama* plays an important role in counteracting depression and sadness. It is both a state of being to strive for and one to rest within. And it has everything to do with being comfortable inside the skin you inhabit. It is the one word I reminded myself of during my entire healing journey, through my divorce and cancer over these last two years. It began with trauma, but along the way it transformed into satisfaction.

SANTOSHA MEANS 'CONTENTMENT.' What appears to be the easiest of these ten yogic codes is perhaps the most challenging to implement. *Santosha* is a state of mind and ease in the body in which, regardless of external situations, you release a deep exhale and say to yourself, 'I'm OK with all of this.' While seemingly different from the other nine codes, contentment takes practice too. We have to learn to be easy with ourselves.

In the *Yoga Sutra* contentment leads to unexcelled joy, whereas the *Darshana Upanishad* expresses it as a delight no matter what happens to you. *Santosha* is expressed as such in the *Mahābhārata*: "Contentment is supreme joy. There is nothing higher than satisfaction. It is complete in itself."

This is the paradox of our species: we have everything we need to survive while we crave for more. This craving leads to incredible insights and life-changing technologies. The shadow side, however, is that we never feel complete, never quite at home within our bodies. The evolutionary rift between our social lives and the interior world of emotions has carved a chasm that persists for a lifetime if left unaddressed. That's why *santosha* is a discipline, a state of being to be worked on, fought for and achieved. Contentment is in no way natural to us. We have to develop it, and then, like any shift in brain mapping, it becomes a state of being that we are grateful for.

Contentment is a low arousal but highly positive emotion marked by feelings of satisfaction, safety and inner peace. The feeling of being wrapped in your lover after sex; watching a child glide down a slide unaccompanied for the first time; closing the last page of a good book and sighing. Contentment is directly related to the CARE system, which provides maternal and parental care as well as nurturance. In its evolutionary biological origins, contentment is rooted in positive emotional bonding mammals and other animals display with their mother/parent figure. This bonding soothes and comforts the baby.

Babies and small children do not have a sufficiently developed prefrontal cortex to modulate their own distressing feelings and emotions. For this they rely upon the physical closeness of their mother to provide calming nurturance. Studies have shown that babies as young as three days old can differentiate the sound of their mother's voice from that of other women, and will respond accordingly. A mixture of hearing her voice and the release of prolactin in her milk provides the calming satisfaction they crave when they cannot verbally express desires.

Consider the opposite: the brain's PANIC system is activated in babies separated from their mothers. These instinctual primitive emotions are also triggered in adults when away from loved ones, or when we experience loss. Being alone is painful. We are social animals who need others, yet we have also (hopefully) been nurtured and healed from emotional panic in our past. We know what loneliness feels like and try to avoid it. There are damaging means of going about this: drug addiction, violence, cynicism, suicide. And then there is meditation and yoga, two practices helping one feel at home.

When a baby's needs are satisfied, contentment arises. Jaak Panksepp explains this emotional process and the origins of how we feel contentment on a biological basis. "Subjective feelings in the human infant would include panic/distress when separation occurs, and contentment/comfort when in contact with the caregiver."

Contentment and tranquility are powerful goals in nearly every religious and spiritual tradition. These feelings are rooted in our evolutionary development. Awareness of mortality provides the motivation for this ultimate quest in achieving emotional security. Putting our trust in something or someone greater than ourselves is at the foundation of numerous traditions. Perhaps this interdependence with our parents leads to the quest of something 'other' for comfort later in life. This goes beyond our mission for survival and exposes us to an innate drive for thriving. Of course, that drive sets us up for disappointment when we do not achieve our goals, but, as stated, it keeps us moving forward individually and culturally. What we can change. What we cannot. The difference between.

The biological origins of contentment are rooted in the extended brain system involving the cingulate gyrus, which mediates and soothes separation distress in infants. This system has a long evolutionary history in the perception of physical pain, providing evidence as to why separation from others is perceived similarly to pain and panic. We have intense evolutionary origins making us afraid of being alone. In this aloneness we are afforded the opportunity to connect with our deepest spiritual practice. What seems like poison is medicine. When the bottom drops out from underneath you, you find out who you really are.

THAT IS, QUITE LITERALLY, the metaphor that changed my life. For years I had seen the writings of American Buddhist nun Pema Chödrön on bookshelves, quotes of hers posted on friends' walls. It was not until going through a divorce that I finally purchased a few of those books, boasting titles that pique your interest as well as make you wonder if you really want to open to page one: *When Things Fall Apart* and *The Places That Scare You.*

What I had expected to be trauma care turned out to be designed for everyday living. True, the teachings are especially potent when going through tough times. Yet in a strange way those are not the hurts that define our character. They help in shaping and molding us, but it is the small upsets, the little things collecting and accumulating, simmering and festering, that drive us to the edge of our emotional limits. Personally I deal with tragedies better than those little gnats buzzing in my ear. Divorce and cancer both stung. Once I put them into perspective—a hard stretch is ahead, but I'll learn a lot in the process and hopefully emerge stronger—I put my head down and did the work. This work is excellent for dealing with our most stubborn neural pathways and ways of life.

This is not an easy path, mind you. One of the most telling phrases comes from Chödrön's teacher, Chögyam Trungpa: smile at fear. Instead of avoiding those places that frighten you, or attempting to justify them as some form of punishment or karma, you develop a relationship with your fears. Trungpa, taking cue from a long history of Buddhist thought, rejects the notion of a divine savior. You yourself, he writes, have to experience the totality of your own suffering and pain. Only then will you understand the nuanced complexity of who you are. This is the road leading to liberation. There are no shortcuts.

You also cannot only chase what makes you happy. The clarion call of the modern positive-only psychology movement has long had detractors. As psychotherapist Mark Epstein writes, "Questioned some years after his enlightenment by a local prince about his penchant for delivering bad news, Buddha said that he could no longer abide by the traditional Sanskrit principle of saying only what was true and pleasant."

Sitting with loneliness, accepting it as a way to find inner peace and cultivate a calm resolve in the face of great panic, resides at the heart of the Tibetan Buddhist meditation practice of *tonglen*. *Tonglen* means 'giving and taking,' undertaken in hopes of creating altruism between you and all living creatures. By diving into the heart of suffering, you understand that all others around you also suffer. Reasons for suffering vary, but it is human to be victimized by thoughts, emotions and expectations. Instead of becoming angry at the world for not being what you want it to be, or turning to a force outside of yourself in hopes that it will 'save' you, you take responsibility for how you act and react to everything you experience. You develop a life in which you treat every person as you would want to be treated, the soul of most every religious tradition throughout recorded history. The world will never be perfect or ideal, given how many different and often conflicting ideas of perfection we have. The practice becomes about being content with imperfections. As Joseph Campbell remarked, it is the Christ on the cross that we truly love: the imperfect man who tried his hardest, not the infallible son of a deity.

The techniques practiced in yoga—meditation, breathing techniques, inquisitive self-reflection—have the ability to change how we act and react. Richard J. Davidson's research confirms this, as we discovered in Chapter Seven. Meditating on different emotions has the capacity of changing our brain maps in different ways. One of the most surprising findings of his work, however, involves how we express ourselves outwardly.

It has long been known that our internal state affects how we appear to others—our posture, facial expressions and general attitude. We also know that social triggers affect our outlook. One study measured people's political views while near a researcher standing next to a garbage can laced with fart spray. Those who filled out a survey near a recently sprayed area were more conservative than those not afflicted by the scent. We are not fixed creatures; our surroundings alter our philosophy and actions. Something as simple as smell has the potential to change our outlook without our being consciously aware of it.

Davidson wanted to know if facial expressions alter our inner state. He devised an ingenious study with women electively undergoing Botox treatments, which paralyzes their corrugator muscle. This muscle is important in expressing sadness and anger. Turns out that these women had a slower response time to stimuli by a quarter-second—a blink of an eye, but an eternity in cognitive neuroscience. Because they had paralyzed part of their facial muscles, their brains were receiving signals more slowly, stunting their emotional responses. In the quest for beauty—in the avoidance of the pain of aging—these women sacrificed their most important neural connection: being in touch with their feelings. If we're avoiding the places that scare us this fear and grief will eventually visit us in unpleasant ways. In all my years of research I've never read one study championing the benefits of suppression.

Once we become content with our situation we can experience the ecstatic mindsets of the mystics we quote and emulate. This does not mean *santosha* becomes a static condition. It is a perpetual practice. Like with any discipline, over time it begins to feel natural. We strengthen our emotions like we gain muscle with continued training. Emotional fortitude generally leads to a more positive and joyous outlook. Neuropsychologist Rick Hanson elaborates on how to rewire our brain from past traumatic experiences, as well as how to deprogram a brain always in reactive mode.

"Taking in the good draws you out of reactive episodes and strengthens the response capacities of your brain. As you weave an underlying sense of strength and wellbeing into yourself, your happiness becomes increasingly unconditional, less and less based on external conditions. Remarkably, the experiences of peace, contentment, and love that are important aims for a good life are also powerful methods for achieving it."

Our brains are losing the ability to relax and find peace in our technologically oriented social media-dominated society. The recent yoga surge in America appears to be a reflex to distraction. Still, inattention is a demon haunting us at every turn. To this day I'm shocked when students pull out their cell phone during class. In fact, certain studios in Los Angeles take no issue with this sort of behavior, and I've been in classes where teachers allow it. One cannot reap the benefits of a system designed for attention and awareness if they cannot unplug for an hour or ninety minutes. You'll always be ripped from the moment, never attentive to what's right in front of you.

Contentment requires the development of positive and focused feelings of inner control. When nurture meets play we feel a higher quality relationship with our emotions. When oxytocin mixes with small amounts of dopamine, contentment appears. Author and yoga teacher Mathew Remski points out that contentment is always available if we allow the simple pleasures of what seems commonplace to unfold naturally. "Many of us have grown too far away from our precognitive skill for trance in childhood. We used to spend hours on the grass gazing at the sky. We knew contentment and somehow we unlearned it. We became busy."

A beautiful image. And for most of us one that takes work. I've long avoided discussing what is and isn't yoga. Yoga has, as we began this book stating, meant many things to many people. But one thing we know for certain: yoga doesn't just happen. It is a discipline that requires patience and practice. That practice matters most off the mat, away from the soothing music, the incense, the soft voice of your favorite instructor, the post-Savasana bliss. There is another, deeper bliss possible when one lives for the greatest good in everyone. It's not an easy path. But in my estimation, nothing could be more worthwhile. Nothing matters more to the world we all inhabit together today.

ABOUT THE AUTHOR

Derek Beres has devoted his life to exposing people to international music, yoga, mythology, and global cultures as a means of creating better individuals and a more informed society. A multi-faceted journalist, DJ, speaker, and yoga instructor, he is the creator of Flow Play, an innovative Vinyasa-based class that fuses yoga, music, and neuroscience, offered nationally at Equinox Fitness. He is also the creator of Warrior Training, a forthcoming interval- and strength-training program for yoga and beyond.

Derek has contributed to dozens of magazines and websites regarding the traditional and digital realms of global music, religion, yoga, and health, including *Women's Health*, *Yoga Journal*, National Geographic, *Rolling Stone Middle East*, *Departures*, AOL and MTV. He worked as the Managing Editor of *Global Rhythm* magazine, and currently writes a weekly column for Big Think, 21st Century Spirituality. *The Warrior's Path* is his seventh book.

He is one half of global music producers EarthRise SoundSystem, which creates innovative contexts for 21st century music and cultures to be explored. Based in Los Angeles, he is on the teacher training faculty at Yogis Anonymous in Santa Monica and Strala Yoga in New York City. He also served as the Creative Director of the Tadasana Festival of Yoga & Music. Derek has been featured in the *NY Times*, *LA Times*, *People*, *Self*, *Shape*, *Fitness*, *Glamour*, *Yoga Journal*, *Boston Globe*, *Newsday*, NBC Weekend Today, ABC Eyewitness News, Fox Business, BBC, KTLA, NY1, MTV, NPR, and PRI.

For more information please visit derekberes.com.

Made in the USA
Charleston, SC
24 August 2014